Primary healthca
South Asian popu...
meeting the challenges

Edited by
Shahid Ali

*Director of Research and Development and Senior Clinical
Research Fellow
Research and Development Unit
Bradford South and West Primary Care Trust*

and

Karl Atkin

*Director of Primary Care Research and Senior Lecturer
Centre for Research in Primary Care
University of Leeds*

Radcliffe Medical Press

Radcliffe Medical Press Ltd
18 Marcham Road
Abingdon
Oxon OX14 1AA
United Kingdom

www.radcliffe-oxford.com
The Radcliffe Medical Press electronic catalogue and online ordering facility.
Direct sales to anywhere in the world.

British Library Cataloguing in Publication Data

A catalogue record for this book is available from the British Library.

ISBN 1 85775 820 X

Typeset by Aarontype Ltd, Easton, Bristol
Printed and bound by TJ International Ltd, Padstow, Cornwall

For Faraaz and Shiraaz (SA)
For Florence and Kris (KA)

Contents

Foreword

This is a book that challenges any existing complacency about the quality of healthcare offered to South Asian populations. It goes much further by questioning the quality of the care actually provided to this often very under-served population whose health problems are frequently exacerbated by their degree of social and economic deprivation. Like any stimulating and well-written book, the authors inform, challenge and occasionally irritate the reader: I experienced all three!

The book is written for a broad audience who have an interest or direct involvement in this important subject area and in my opinion will appeal to leaders, clinicians, nursing staff, managers, and the wider primary care community.

Research, analysis and commentary are essential, but if South Asian people are to benefit from better services and improved care, then research in particular must be integrated with dissemination and development. This is a responsibility of all those working in the area, particularly since the book is presented at a time when radical changes in the NHS are in progress. This provides an excellent opportunity, as the authors argue, to improve healthcare to the South Asian Population, through Primary Care Trusts (locally based and with virtually the whole local NHS budget and the involvement of community-based clinicians), National Service Frameworks (addressing all aspects of anticipatory care, which of course includes prevention), Local Strategic Partnerships (that focus on both partnership working and community development) and not least a large increase in NHS funding (a considerable part of which is for general practice-based teams to deliver probably the largest quality-based contract attempted anywhere in the world). These represent a real commitment to promoting equality.

The NHS Plan, for example, is a ten-year programme and not a short-term approach. And many of the targets established by Department of Health priorities are relevant to addressing the inequity of opportunity and service that the book articulates so well. The National Service Frameworks establish key priorities as do government policies to address health inequalities. At the time of going to print there is also a Department of Health push to explore how to improve choice, responsiveness and equity in health and social care – a national and local consultation which includes very specifically the black and minority ethnic population. Similarly, the DoH has launched a consultation on mental health services for black and minority ethnic communities: *Delivering Racial Equality*.

You see the book did engage me, which is the hallmark of a good read. I most certainly recommend it, as I am sure it will engage you too. Inequity and inequality must be rigorously challenged and addressed. This book does that.

David Colin-Thomé
National Clinical Director of Primary Care
Department of Health
General Practitioner, Runcorn
November 2004

List of contributors

Martin Commander, Consultant Psychiatrist, Birmingham and Solihull Mental Health NHS Trust, Birmingham

Stephen Harrison, Professor of Social Policy, Department of Applied Social Science, University of Manchester, Manchester

Philip Heywood, Professor of Primary Care Development, Academic Unit of Primary Care, University of Leeds, Leeds

Rukshana Kapasi, Management Consultant, SILKAP Consultants, Wembley

Dee Kyle, Director of Public Health, Bradford South and West Primary Care Trust, Bradford

Timothy Milewa, Lecturer in Sociology, Brunel Health Services Research Collaboration, Centre for the Study of Health, Department of Human Sciences, Brunel University, Uxbridge

Dinesh Nagi, Consultant Physician in Diabetes/Endocrinology, Pinderfields General Hospital, Wakefield

James Nazroo, Senior Lecturer in Sociology, Department of Epidemiology and Public Health, University College London, London

Sashi Sashidharan, Professor of Community Psychiatry and Medical Director, Birmingham and Solihull Mental Health NHS Trust, Birmingham

Acknowledgements

Professor Waqar IU Ahmad provided encouragement and guidance during the initial discussions about the content of the book. We would also like to thank individuals from Bradford primary care trusts, who have provided valuable advice during the preparation of this manuscript, as well as our colleagues at the Centre for Research in Primary Care for their ongoing support and advice. Hazel Blackburn provided considerable help in preparing the final manuscript.

Finally, we would like to thank Paula Moran at Radcliffe Medical Press for her support and patience.

PART 1

Ethnicity and primary care

CHAPTER 1

Meeting the challenges

Karl Atkin and Shahid Ali

It is now a decade since United Kingdom (UK) healthcare policy recognised the 'particular care needs' of minority ethnic populations.[1] Primary care, although part of these broad debates, has only recently merited special attention. This is perhaps surprising, given the increasing importance of primary care to healthcare delivery in the UK.[2] Current changes give primary care trusts (PCTs) the opportunity to commission services in accordance with the needs of local populations. In doing so, PCTs are supported by priorities established by the various National Service Frameworks (NFSs) and quality guarantees assured through the process of clinical governance, which aim to improve the quality of primary care available to UK citizens. The primary care agenda, however, has been slow to reflect the more general principle, now well established, of providing accessible care appropriate to the needs of minority ethnic populations.[3] South Asian populations are, of course, an important part of these debates and like many other health professionals, those working in primary care can sometimes be confused about how best to engage with such populations. At best, this means the perspectives and needs of South Asian people do not adequately inform service delivery.[4] At worst, it means service support is informed by racist myths and stereotypes.[5]

South Asian populations represent the largest minority ethnic community in the UK, are subject to considerable material inequalities, have high rates of chronic disease, and find it difficult to access healthcare services appropriate to their needs.[6] For example, according to 1997 figures, the average weekly household income for Bangladeshi families was £196. The figure was not much higher for Pakistani families (£203). The weekly average for the general population was over £100 higher at £343.[7] South Asian populations are also more likely to live in poor housing stock, without basic amenities such as central heating and washing machines.[7] Perhaps not surprisingly, given this material disadvantage, Bangladeshi and Pakistani individuals are twice as likely to report long-standing health problems as the general population and South Asian groups have higher rates of diabetes and heart disease than any other ethnic grouping.[8] Further, South Asian populations often experience difficulties in accessing public services and when they do, they find themselves subject to inappropriate service support that is unable to accommodate diversity and difference.[6]

Provision of primary healthcare occurs within this broader context and the current reorganisation of services has to engage with increasing evidence of health inequalities as well as difficulties of access and insensitive service provision to South Asian populations. This book, by discussing these issues, aims to offer practitioners and managers a broad introduction to the difficulties of providing good quality primary healthcare provision to South Asian populations. In doing so, it examines issues such as institutional racism and equal opportunities in relation to the more generic issues raised by organisation and delivery of care. The book, however, is not simply about offering an analysis of the problems of offering equitable and appropriate primary healthcare. By simply highlighting the negative consequences of service provision we are in danger of, in the words of Zygmunt Bauman, 'leaving a waste ground devoid of meaning',[9] which does little to transform policy and practice. This is why the book also proposes possible solutions for overcoming these problems, by focusing on practical examples of partnership working and user involvement, identifying instances of good practices and emphasising the importance of empowerment. Clinical governance, for example, provides a potential lever for change and can help ensure 'ethnicity and health' is placed on the primary healthcare agenda. Similarly, Department of Health rhetoric on user involvement can be used to ensure health commissioners listen to the experience of local communities and ensure their voice informs the process of service delivery. More broadly, amendments to the Race Relations Act and the Commission for Racial Equality's intent to establish performance management indicators to ensure health and social care agencies comply with the provision of the Act offer another important potential for change.[10]

Poor quality care, discrimination and disadvantage, therefore, are not inevitable and there are plenty of opportunities to ensure the healthcare needs of South Asian populations are central to agenda informing primary healthcare. This book makes its own modest contribution to these debates and should initiate a discussion among those working in primary care about how best to meet the needs of South Asian people.

Outline of the book

The book is in four parts. Part 1 sets the scene by outlining the broad themes informing our present understanding of ethnicity and primary care. First, it explores the theoretical context mediating our current understanding of ethnicity and health before focusing on the concerns that inform the current organisation and delivery of primary care. Part 2 uses specific policy examples, such as clinical governance, user involvement and partnership, to explore primary care organisations' relationship to South Asian populations. Part 3, adopts a different approach and presents condition-specific case studies – coronary heart disease, mental health and diabetes – which reflect current National Health Service (NHS) priorities. Part 4 offers a conclusion that explores the specific implications of 'what we know' for the future development of primary healthcare. In doing so, it discusses how current changes in the organisation of primary care and our understanding of the healthcare needs of South Asian populations can be used to improve service support.

The book begins with an introduction to institutional racism and reviews current theoretical developments in how we make sense of discrimination and difference. In doing so, it outlines themes that underpin the analysis offered by the other chapters in this volume. All the chapters, for example, explore the disadvantages experienced by South Asian communities and the difficulties facing primary healthcare agencies in their attempts to tackle this disadvantage. In doing so, the authors also offer possible solutions aimed at overcoming these problems and thereby provide opportunities for a more equitable and accessible primary care which meets the needs of South Asian people. However, to fully exploit the insights offered by these chapters, theoretical reconciliation is required. This is important for three reasons. First, debates about primary healthcare should not be isolated from the more mainstream discussion informing our understanding of ethnicity. Many of the issues facing primary care as it struggles to make sense of disadvantage and diversity are generic problems facing all public services. It is important not to reinvent the wheel and to learn from the experience of others who have tried to make sense of these issues. Second – and as a consequence of this failure to engage with these mainstream debates – discussions about South Asian populations and primary care often present health professionals with uncontextualised accounts that do not reflect the diversity and complexity of people's experience. Such approaches can lead to simplistic and unsophisticated responses that perhaps ironically perpetuate disadvantage and discrimination by encouraging ill-advised policy and practice developments. Third, there is a need to empower primary care professionals by providing them with a critical understanding that enables them to tackle, rather than be overwhelmed by, the problems of providing healthcare in a multi-ethnic society. In offering a preliminary understanding of the theoretical themes informing discussions about healthcare for minority ethnic groups, Chapter 2 aims to provide primary care professionals with the confidence to engage with these often complex and politically charged debates.

The chapter by Philip Heywood considers the organisation and delivery of primary care. In doing so, he refines our focus and outlines the specific remit of primary care and how it relates to the needs of South Asian populations. He begins by examining the role of equal opportunities within the changing structure of primary care, before exploring the implications, challenges and opportunities faced by those working in primary care as they attempt to offer equitable and sensitive healthcare. Just as mainstream debates about ethnicity and health should inform primary care development, discussions about ethnicity and health must also engage with the current changes occurring in primary care.

The second part of the book begins to engage with the specifics of service delivery and focuses on three broad policy concerns central to the Department of Health's strategy of improving health outcomes. Stephen Harrison uses his chapter to explore how clinical governance can be adopted as a lever of change to ensure primary care engages with ethnicity and health. Taking this as his starting point, he offers some conceptual clarity on this often confusing subject before examining the policy and practice issues suggested by the implementation of clinical governance. A particular concern is how PCTs make sense of clinical governance within the wider context of NSFs and how this, in turn, can be used to improve equity. Harrison concludes, however, that the debate about clinical governance represents a double-edged sword and although offering benefits for the individual healthcare of South Asian patients, it also raises the potential for inhibiting broader discussions about inequalities. This offers a timely reminder that policy and practice are not enacted in a straightforward way, but offer contradiction and compromise, which create both opportunities and dangers for South Asian populations. Strategy and struggle are therefore required, and in this respect empowerment is key in ensuring the needs of South Asian populations appropriately inform the primary healthcare agenda.

Timothy Milewa and Rukshana Kapasi follow up these issues and explore the prospects of user involvement in primary care. The Department of Health has placed considerable emphasis on patient and public involvement in recent years, but healthcare agencies have had difficultly when engaging with South Asian populations. As Milewa and Kapasi point out, communication, cultural differences and the attitudes of health professionals can sometimes mitigate against the involvement of South Asian users. They then offer empirical evidence on recent attempts by PCTs to involve South Asian people in primary care and go on to identify key issues that facilitate successful public involvement among minority ethnic groups. Part 2 ends with Dee Kyle offering a specific case study looking at how partnership with local populations can improve healthcare for South Asian people. Kyle offers a practitioner's account. Achieving partnership, as we shall see, is a complex and often frustrating process for health professionals. The chapter reminds us about the realities of service delivery and the dilemmas facing those working in primary care as they struggle to offer support that meets the needs of South Asian populations. Nonetheless, it concludes that curiosity, empathy and respect are key to building productive partnerships.

Part 3 offers evidence on specific disease examples which reflect NSF priorities. Each author approaches their example in a different way, yet all are able to develop an evidence base from which they are able to offer advice on how to improve healthcare for South Asian people. James Nazroo discusses coronary heart disease among South Asian communities and makes sense of ethnic inequalities by using secondary data analysis to explore the implications of genetic risk, lifestyle, culture, material disadvantage and racism on heart disease. In doing so, his analysis gives empirical expression to several themes raised in Chapter 2. By emphasising the importance of not treating South Asian populations as a homogeneous group, he illustrates how policy and practice have to accommodate diversity and difference. He also suggests that socio-economic position is equally as important as ethnicity in explaining higher rates of coronary heart disease among South Asian populations. Sashi Sashidharan and Martin Commander specifically demonstrate the importance of grounding empirical analysis in the broader themes of disadvantage and focus on the psychiatric experiences of South Asian populations. They argue that the current policy and practice framework in which judgements are made about the mental health needs of South Asian people needs to be critically assessed: rejecting simplistic cultural explanations and accommodating ideas such as disadvantage, discrimination and dislocation. The final chapter in Part 3 explores diabetes. Diabetes is a particular health problem facing South Asian populations and, as Dinesh Nagi demonstrates, is three to four times more common than in the general population. This chapter, by offering a thematic review of research evidence, focuses on the epidemiology, aetiology and the socio-economic consequences of diabetes for South Asian people. In doing so, it presents a detailed and comprehensive evidence base which explains differences in outcomes between South Asian and European populations. This is then used as a basis to understanding and overcoming barriers to good quality care in primary care.

Part 4 offers a discussion and makes sense of the various themes explored by the book. In doing so, we emphasise how better knowledge can lead to better care and better outcomes within the context of primary care policy and practice. By reviewing the mix of theoretical and empirical debates raised by the authors, this final chapter looks at how primary healthcare can efficiently meet the needs of an ethnically and culturally diverse society. It specifically emphasises the importance of exploiting our existing evidence base and theoretical understanding to meet the challenges of offering accessible and appropriate primary healthcare to South Asian populations as well as outlining the value of learning from good practice.

References

1   Department of Health (1989) *Caring for People: community care in the next decade and beyond.* Cmnd. 849. HMSO, London.
2   Department of Health (2000) *The NHS Plan.* HMSO, London.
3   Ahmad WIU (2000) Introduction. In: Ahmad WIU (ed) *Ethnicity, Disability and Chronic Illness.* Open University Press, Buckingham.
4   Mason D (2000) *Race and Ethnicity in Modern Britain.* Oxford University Press, Oxford.
5   Law I (1996) *Racism, Ethnicity and Social Policy.* Harvester Wheatsheaf, Brighton.
6   Atkin K (2003) Health care in South Asian populations: making sense of policy and practice. In: Sayyid B and Ali N (eds) *South Asian Populations in the UK.* Hurst, London.
7   Modood T, Bethould R, Lakey J *et al.* (1997) *Ethnic Minorities in Britain.* Social Policy Studies Institute, London.
8   Nazroo J (1996) *Health of Ethnic Minorities.* Policy Studies Institute, London.
9   Bauman Z (1992) *Intimations of Post Modernity.* Routledge, London.
10   Commission for Racial Equality (2003) *Stakeholder Strategy Consultation: health and social care.* CRE, London.

CHAPTER 2

Institutional racism, policy and practice

Karl Atkin

The primary care agenda, as we have seen, has been slow to provide accessible care appropriate to the needs of minority ethnic populations and rarely engages with broader debates about ethnicity and health. In response to this and to enable those working in primary care to reflect on these issues, this opening chapter establishes the theoretical context in which we make sense of the inequalities experienced by South Asian populations. We begin by discussing institutional racism and explore its value to making sense of the disadvantages faced by minority ethnic groups in relation to healthcare. Institutional racism has recently become a fashionable term, used to explain the failings of public institutions to respond to the needs of minority ethnic populations living in the UK.[1] Nonetheless, in becoming fashionable the term risks becoming little more than a 'buzz' word of little or no analytical value. To recapture the meaning of institutional racism, the chapter breaks down the concept into its various themes and offers empirical examples to establish its validity. We then further sensitise the idea of institutional racism by critically evaluating what we mean by 'ethnicity' and in particular exploring its purpose as an explanatory variable in understanding disadvantage and discrimination. The chapter ends by emphasising the importance of using our awareness and knowledge of racism to transform policy and practice. As we shall see, focusing on the needs of South Asian populations is not the same as responding to these needs. Often there is a gap between our understanding of the issues and our willingness to act on their implications to improve service delivery.[2,3] This will be a recurring theme throughout the book.

Institutional racism, South Asian populations and primary healthcare

'Institutional racism' has recently entered popular consciousness, being used regularly in the media, mentioned in politicians' speeches and offered as a knowing explanation, as British public services struggle to respond to the needs of an ethnically diverse society. This interest can be attributed directly to the Macpherson inquiry into the death of Steven Lawrence, which concluded that UK organisations, including health and social care agencies, were institutionally racist. Such sentiments became embodied in law with the introduction in April 2001 of amendments to the 1976 Race Relations Act, which made statutory agencies responsible for promoting equal opportunities and identifying and tackling institutional racism within their organisation. As a consequence of the Act, all public bodies, for example, are required to have race equality strategies in place. The Commission for Racial Equality (CRE) sought to further clarify the issue by stating its intent to develop a strategy to ensure health and social care agencies take institutional racism seriously and comply with the changes in their legal responsibilities.[4] Primary Care Trusts are accorded special attention in the CRE's strategy, perhaps reflecting the status as developing organisations with little previous experience in providing equitable services that meet the needs of minority ethnic populations.

   Despite this recent policy interest, institutional racism is not a new idea and was first introduced over 20 years ago.[5] Since then, institutional racism has gradually emerged as an extremely helpful and productive idea in making sense of health inequalities as well as inappropriate and inaccessible service provision.[6] Institutional racism is often called camouflaged racism, meaning that it is not immediately obvious but embedded in the taken-for-granted assumptions informing organisation practices. It occurs when the policies of an institution lead to discriminatory outcomes for minority ethnic populations, irrespective of the motives of individual employees of that institution.[7] Institutional racism, in effect, is the uncritical application of policies and procedures that ignore the needs of an ethnically diverse society.[8] Such practices, by default, favour the majority white population, who are assumed to represent the 'norm' around which service delivery becomes organised.[9] Service users, for example, are assumed to have Western attitudes, priorities, expectations and values; act according to Western ways; speak English and understand the organisation of public services.[10]

   Analytically, institutional racism combines two specific themes which explain the response of health and social care agencies to the needs of South Asian populations. First, potential differences in need between South Asian people and the general population are disregarded as 'one service' is assumed to 'fit' all. Second, when difference is recognised, it is done in such a way as to misrepresent the needs of South Asian populations, thereby encouraging inappropriate policy and practice responses.

Constructing need: ignoring difference and diversity

Perhaps the heart of the problem, and fundamental to our understanding of institutional racism, is the idea that the same service for all equates with an equal service for all.[2] This can be a consequence of genuine ignorance, a deliberate failure to engage with difference, or of being so overwhelmed by the difficulties of providing care to a multi-ethnic population that providing a generic service is seen as the easiest option. The outcome, however, is the same and services come to obscure their failures to meet the needs of minority ethnic people by assuming they treat everyone the same. In reality this means that services are organised, by default, according to a 'white norm' and do not recognise difference and diversity.[6] There is an underlying assumption that policies, procedures and practices are equally appropriate for everyone.[11] Such practices legitimise non recognition of the care needs of minority ethnic communities and disregard the specific dietary, linguistic and cultural needs of South Asian populations.[7]

The inability of the NHS to provide adequate support of those whose first language is not English is the most obvious example of this[12] and has particular implications for primary care, where it is extremely difficult to gain access to appropriate language support.[13] It is worth exploring this further as a lack of language support illustrates the complex nature of institutional racism and its consequences for minority ethnic populations.[14] In the first instance, interpreters are often in short supply and difficult to get hold of, especially in primary care settings.[12] This is why, when a person cannot speak English, family members are sometimes used as interpreters and, although acceptable to some people, others object to the practice.[15] In some cases young children are required to act as interpreters of complex medical information, often about sensitive or potentially embarrassing issues.[16] This is unfair to both the child and the person they are expected to interpret for. Other family members point to the problems they faced in simultaneously translating distressing information to a close relative and coming to terms with it themselves. Family members also speak of the difficulties in deciding how much they should tell their non-English speaking relatives: often they wanted to 'protect them' from information deemed upsetting. This, however, often left the relative without important information about their health; information important for understanding, coping and caring as well as for deciding what course of action to take.[16] In other cases, patients did not want their health problem shared with other family members, and would have preferred a confidential consultation in which they could discuss their concerns.[12] They felt, however, that this was not an option because of the lack of language support and therefore believed they had no alternative but to accept family support.[17]

Difficulties still occur when interpreters are used.[18] Most interpreters, for example, have little specialist knowledge and face difficulties in interpreting clinical information and procedures, sometimes with unfortunate consequences. This means that patients often gain misleading and erroneous information about their illness or care options.[15] Patients and their families also point to the problems of communicating through a third party. This, they felt, made it difficult to ask questions and more generally take part in a discussion with health professionals. Often, for example, the discussion is limited to closed questions rather than more open exploration of the issues. Not surprisingly, patients and their families express dissatisfaction with the process.[17,18] Many practitioners, for their part, share these concerns about the shortfalls in interpreting services. For example, interpreters are often not available or else difficult to organise. Those working in primary care face particular difficulties as the unpredictable nature of some of their work means they often do not know which patients will turn up in the consulting room.[13] Practitioners also questioned interpreters' skills as well as their own competence in working with interpreters.[16] For these reasons, many health professionals prefer to use family members because it provides them flexibility,[15] although as we have seen this is sometimes not the ideal option for the patient.

The difficulties of providing adequate language support in primary care create barriers to effective communication and make it difficult to respond to and meet the healthcare needs of South Asian populations.[12] Barriers to communications, however, are more than language specific and evoke cultural differences,[19] particularly since ethnic and cultural misunderstandings, myths and stereotypes can undermine the communication process. Most healthcare professionals, for example, feel ill-equipped to respond to cultural differences and rarely appropriately understand the lifestyles, social customs and religious practices of people from ethnic minority groups.[16] Making sense of this introduces our second theme: misrepresenting the healthcare needs of minority ethnic populations.

Misrepresenting the healthcare needs of South Asian populations

When health and social care agencies do recognise the differences of South Asian populations, it is often to the disadvantage of such populations. There are several ways in which this is done. Sometimes it is the consequence of ill-informed views about the cause of problems presented by South Asian populations; at other times it is the use of inappropriate myths and stereotypes, which although purporting to explain the behaviour and beliefs of South Asian populations, do little more than misrepresent their experience (see Parekh, 2000 for a discussion of these issues).[20]

To begin with, health and social services often identify South Asian health and social 'problems' as arising from cultural practices.[19] This results in service organisations blaming minority ethnic communities for the problems they experience.[21] Minority ethnic people, for example, are frequently characterised as in some way to blame for their own needs because of deviant, unsatisfactory and pathological lifestyles.[22] This has led some people to observe that in health matters, minority ethnic populations suffer twice: once because of the actual health problem and second because their health problems are then turned against them.[23] Indeed there is a history of defining health problems faced by South Asian populations in terms of cultural deficits where a shift towards a 'Western' lifestyle is offered as the main solution to their problems; examples include the discussions on maternity and child health[24] and diet and rickets.[25]

Such views become embedded in the views of front-line practitioners working in health and social services; South Asian people become seen as a problem.[25] Practitioners working in local authorities often list South Asian people as 'high-risk' clients, 'unco-operative' and 'difficult to work with'. Similarly, evidence suggests that racism within the NHS affects minority ethnic people with common stereotypes portraying them as 'calling out doctors unnecessarily', 'being trivial complainers' and 'time wasters'.[2] These attitudes can deprive South Asian people of their rights to services, especially since health and social service professionals exercise considerable discretion in their day-to-day work.[26]

A more complex example of how the healthcare needs of South Asian populations become misrepresented through the pathologising of cultural practices concerns how impairment, and more generally 'poor birth outcome', become attributed to consanguineous marriages.[22] Health professionals, for example, often related thalassaemia major among Pakistani families to consanguineous marriages and therefore considered it to be self-inflicted and located in these communities, and so presumed cultural and biological pathology.[15,27] The relationship between consanguineous marriage and the incidence of impairment and poor health is, of course, complex.[22] In some cases, marrying a first cousin can increase a family's risk of giving birth to a disabled or chronically ill child, especially if there is a history of certain conditions in the extended family.[28] First-cousin marriage, however, is not the only cause of disability or chronic illness in Pakistani or Bangladeshi families, and there is good evidence to suggest its influence has been overemphasised (see

Ahmad *et al.*, 2000 for a review of the evidence).[22] Such an approach not only carries with it an implicit (and misleading) criticism of Asian cultural practices, thereby creating mistrust between health professionals and their patients,[11] it also misrepresents the origins of ill health and therefore leads to misguided policy approaches.[15] The preoccupation with consanguineous marriage in explaining impairment means other important explanations, such as poverty, poor maternal health, inappropriate housing or inadequate service support, are rarely mentioned. Low socio-economic status, for example, seems far more influential than ethnic origin or cultural difference in explaining ill health among South Asian populations.[29] We also know that poor antenatal and postnatal care are more likely to explain impairment and ill health in South Asian families than cultural practices.[30]

An overemphasis on the consequences of first-cousin marriages, at the expense of other more relevant explanations, offers a straightforward example of institutional racism. Misrepresentation of South Asian beliefs and values, however, has another dimension. As part of this preoccupation with culture, minority ethnic groups also have to contend with inappropriate generalisations of cultural practices and the use of simplistic explanations to explain their behaviour.[6] Ironically, many of these problems occur because authors want to be helpful and provide explanations that enable health professionals to respond to the needs of a multi-ethnic society. Such explanations, however, tend to present static and one-dimensional views of cultural norms and values, which are devoid of context and allow no room for individual interpretation.[9] They can also create the illusion that they offer a solution to an extremely complex situation.[25] Introductory notes on minority ethnic communities, present in most training material for service practitioners, often follow this pattern. One would not, for instance, attempt to summarise a Western approach to child-rearing practices in one paragraph, yet this is what minority ethnic people are subjected to. Similarly, it is common to see one-page explanations of Muslim, Hindu and Sikh culture, in which patients' beliefs are expected to correspond. Such approaches, however, perpetuate myths and stereotypes that further serve to disadvantage South Asian populations.

A useful example illustrating the dangers of such approaches emerges by exploring provision of prenatal diagnosis. Assumptions held by practitioners can deny families choice, thereby excluding them from decisions about their own and their children's healthcare.[16] Myths, often derived from simplistic accounts of Islamic beliefs, explain why prenatal diagnosis is sometimes withheld from Muslim families. Termination is assumed unacceptable to such families because it is incompatible with Islamic values. The empirical reality, however, is far more complex than this. Like other sections of the UK population,[31] termination is acceptable to some Muslim families but not to others.[15] There is no one Islamic interpretation of the acceptability of termination and families' decision-making process is informed by their own values and beliefs (including their interpretation of Islam), the views of other family members, the role of healthcare professionals and whether they already have a child with the condition.[15] Moreover, people's views can also change over time and a decision taken during one pregnancy might not be the same as one taken in future pregnancies.[16]

Another more general myth that contributes further to our failure to recognise the support needs of South Asian families is the convenient idea that 'they' virtuously 'look after their own'. Health and social care agencies use this as a reason for not planning or providing services for disabled or chronically ill individuals or their families.[19] The assumption that Asian people live in self-supporting, extended family networks is simplistic for a number of reasons (Ahmad, 1993 provides a detailed account of these reasons).[25] Household structures, for example, are changing as well as the expectations that inform family obligations. Indian family structure, with a move to more nuclear households, is beginning to reflect that of the general population and although three-generational households are still common among Pakistani and Bangladeshi families, there are more people who do not live in three-generational households than who do.[32] This, however, is perhaps not the real issue. The assumption that extended Asian families have the necessary material, emotional and social resources to cope with chronic illness with limited professional support is at best misguided and at worst a racist denial of their support needs.[33]

Beyond institutional racism

Institutional racism provides a framework which enables us to make sense of the discrimination and disadvantages faced by minority ethnic groups, as they try and gain access to appropriate healthcare. It allows us to explain why the linguistic, cultural and religious needs of South Asian populations are disregarded by health and social care agencies. Institutional racism also helps us to understand that when difference is recognised by services, it is often to the disadvantage of minority ethnic populations. Providing responsive and equitable service provision for South Asian populations, however, requires us to further 'sensitise' our conception of institutional racism. Two distinct principles – one broadly theoretical, the other more practical – emerge as significant. The first focuses on how we make sense of terms such as ethnicity, differences and diversity. The second is more concerned with how we can translate evidence about the process of disadvantage into improved outcomes for South Asian populations. It is to these we now turn.

Making sense of ethnic differences

Ethnicity is a notoriously difficult concept to define. Previous understandings that classified people according to their country of origin are no longer sustainable, particularly since nearly 40 per cent of what we regard as minority ethnic populations are born in the UK.[32] Consequently, young people are beginning to redefine their identity and adopting such terms as British Muslim or British Asian or even British Indian. Young people are also increasingly using religious affiliations, such as Muslim or Hindu or Sikh, to describe who they are (see Ahmad *et al.*, 2002 for a discussion of these broad issues).[34] This perhaps reflects fundamental differences in how young people and parents make sense of their identity and variations in their broader engagement with British society,[35] although this is not to say that young people are wholly rejecting their parents' identifications. There is considerable continuity in values between the different generations.[34]

   The emergence of these debates highlights diversity both between and within South Asian populations. Little more than a decade ago, it was possible for policy to present South Asian populations as a discrete group. We now recognise differ-ences in both socio-economic positions and cultural values among Indian, Pakistani and Bangladeshi populations[29] (see also Chapter 9). As part of this, we are also beginning to understand the importance of religion in making sense of the lives of South Asian populations.[32] Nor is religion a simple marker of cultural differences. The socio-economic position of Indian Muslims, for example, reveals they have more in common with Pakistani Muslims than Indian populations.[18] Regional identification also emerges as important in explaining ethnic differences, even when people share the same country of origin. In Pakistan, cultural, linguistic and socio-economic differences occur between those people who originate from the Punjab and those who originate form the North-West frontier. Moreover, those who claim Miripui Punjabi heritage represent a cultural and linguistic commun-ity distinct from the rest of the Punjab. Kashmiri identity can also emerge as an important marker of identity for some, rather than allegiance to either Pakistan or India.[36]

In some ways, the multifaceted way in which we have come to understand 'ethnicity' has both disadvantages and advantages as we attempt to tackle dis-advantages and discrimination. Conceptual confusion can sometimes occur and ethnicity can be used to obscure more fundamental differences among populations. At the same time, the complex and shifting nature of ethnicity also provides a use-ful framework in which to explore diversity and differences between and among populations. Ethnicity is not a neutral term and has come to embody language, religion, culture, nationality and a shared heritage.[34] Further, ethnicity has increas-ingly been seen as a political symbol, defining not just exclusion by a powerful majority but also a source of pride and belonging;[20] in other words, a mobilising resource which enables South Asian populations to celebrate their differences and make legitimate demands as UK citizens.[36]

More generally, as part of our concern with diversity, we need also to accept that in some ways minority ethnic populations may not be all that different from the general population.[7] It is, therefore, important to use essentialising notions of ethnicity. Patients with end-stage cancer, for example, articulate many similar concerns, worries and needs, irrespective of ethnicity.[37] This is also reflected in their service needs. Not every problem or difficulty a person encounters as they attempt to gain access to appropriate service delivery can be attributed to their ethnic back-ground. By improving services generally we can often improve support for South Asian populations.[25] The challenge is to know when ethnicity makes a difference and mediates a person's relationship with service support and when it does not. There is increasing evidence that socio-economic status, age and gender are as important as ethnicity in making sense of a person's health and social care needs (see also Chapter 9).[37] Policy and practice need to recognise this and understand how ethnicity relates to other aspects of an individual's identity. Otherwise they will offer solutions on the basis of misguided and mistaken premises. South Asian women, for example, sometimes struggle to convince doctors that their child is seriously ill and find themselves being dismissed as 'neurotic' or 'overprotective'.[15] Lack of language support and assumptions about the passivity of South Asian women contribute to such views. Nonetheless, their treatment is not wholly a consequence of their ethnic background but can be explained by doctors' more general sexist attitudes.[38]

Using evidence to improve policy and practice

In addition to the theoretical concerns outlined above, institutional racism also needs to accommodate more practical issues. Offering an analysis of the problems facing South Asian populations is one thing; doing something about it is another. Accounts of institutional racism tend to focus on the unfair structuring of opportunities.[6] The critical emphasis of the literature is perhaps understandable and has successfully highlighted the negative consequences of racism, marginalisation and unequal treatment.[11] Nonetheless, by constantly highlighting the negative consequences of service provision, we do little to advance thinking and practice.[39] We have accumulated a good deal of evidence outlining the process and outcomes of institutional racism. Policy and practice, however, have been less successful in translating these insights into improvements in service delivery. This is now the challenge facing those working in primary care. We need to understand, for example, more about what constitutes good practice and how such practice can be sustained and replicated in other localities.[9] Future research outlining the difficulties facing South Asian populations is perhaps unhelpful. Research needs to refocus its attention on understanding how services can best meet the needs of South Asian populations by exploring more about how services are delivered and suggesting ways they can be improved (Chapter 6, for example, provides several examples of good practice). As well as defining problems, our growing evidence base must also offer solutions. All the chapters in this volume, for example, use an evidence base to offer potential solutions to improving healthcare outcomes for South Asian people. Without such a commitment to change, service initiatives are not only in danger of wasting valuable public resources but are also in jeopardy of becoming little more than token gestures, leading to increasing disillusionment and estrangement among South Asian populations.[3]

Conclusion

This chapter provides a generic introduction to institutional racism and offers a theoretical framework to help us make sense of the following chapters. This is especially valuable because primary care has been slow to engage with debates about institutional racism. This chapter suggests that the healthcare needs of South Asian populations are either ignored or, if they are recognised, become seen as a problem subject to various stereotypes and myths. This offers an initial starting point in making sense of the experiences of South Asian people living in the UK and in developing accessible and appropriate primary care provision.

At the same time, however, the chapter points out that we need to recognise the complexity of ethnic differences. This means acknowledging differences between and within different ethnic populations as well as accepting that ethnicity is not always the only explanation for disadvantage and discrimination. Ethnic diversity must be understood within a broader context which recognises socioeconomic status, age and gender are equally as important in making sense of a person's health and social care needs.

We also need to ground our understanding of institutional racism in a commitment to improve outcomes for South Asian populations. Using what we know to make improvements in service delivery is a far from straightforward process, and in the past policy and practice have seemed overwhelmed by the difficulties of responding to the needs of South Asian populations. The process of discrimination, although well understood, has not always been used to transform service delivery. Policy and practice, therefore, need to shift their focus and find out more about the principles of good practice. This will ensure that service development can benefit from a better understanding of what works for South Asian populations.

References

1   Macpherson W (1999) *The Stephen Lawrence Inquiry: report of an inquiry by Sir William Macpherson of Cluny.* (Cm 4262-I.) HMSO, London.

2   Atkin K (1996) Race and social policy. In: Lunt N and Coyle D (eds) *Welfare and Policy.* Taylor and Francis, Basingstoke.

3   Mir G and Nocon A (2002) Partnership, advocacy and independence: service principles and the empowerment of minority ethnic people. *Journal of Learning Disabilities.* **6** (2): 153–62.

4   Commission for Racial Equality (2003) *Stakeholder Strategy Consultation: health and social care.* CRE, London.

5   Glasgow D (1980) *The Black Underclass.* Jossey Bass, London.

6   Law I (1996) *Racism, Ethnicity and Social Policy.* Harvester Wheatsheaf, Brighton.

7   Mason D (2000) *Race and Ethnicity in Modern Britain.* Oxford University Press, Oxford.

8   Weller B (1991) Nursing in a multi-cultural world. *Nursing Standard.* **5** (30): 31–2.

9   Atkin K (2003) Health care in South Asian populations: making sense of policy and practice. In: Sayyid B, Ali N and Singh VK (eds) *Asian Nation: postcolonial settlers in Britain.* Hurst, London.

10 Butt J and Mirza K (1996) *Social Care and Black Communities.* HMSO, London.

11 Ahmad WIU (2000) Introduction. In: Ahmad WIU (ed) *Ethnicity, Disability and Chronic Illness.* Open University Press, Buckingham.

12 Robinson M (2001) *Communication and Health in a Multi-ethnic Society.* Policy Press, Bristol.

13 Ali N, Neal R and Atkin K (2003) *Communication between GPs and South Asian Patients: final report to Northern and Yorkshire Regional Health Authority.* Centre for Research in Primary Care, Leeds.

14 Association of London Government (2000) *Sick of Being Excluded: improving the health and care of London's black and minority ethnic communities.* Association of London Government, London.

15 Atkin K, Ahmad WIU and Anionwu E (1998) Screening and counselling for sickle cell disorders and thalassaemia: the experience of parents and health professionals. *Social Science and Medicine.* **47** (11): 1639–51.

16 Anionwu E and Atkin K (2001) *The Politics of Sickle Cell and Thalassaemia.* Open University Press, Buckingham.

17 Bhakta P, Katbamna S and Parker G (2000) South Asian carers' experiences of primary health care teams. In: Ahmad WIU (ed) *Ethnicity, Disability and Chronic Illness.* Open University Press, Buckingham.

18   Chamba R, Hirst M, Lawton D *et al.* (1999) *On the Edge: a national survey of minority ethnic parents caring for a severely disabled child.* Policy Press, Bristol.

19   Walker R and Ahmad WIU (1994) Windows of opportunity in rotting frames: care providers' perspectives on community care. *Critical Social Policy.* **40**: 46–9.

20   Parekh B (2000) *Rethinking multi-culturalism: cultural diversity and political theory.* Palgrave, Basingstoke.

21   Bowler I (1993) They are not the same as us: midwives' stereotypes of South Asian maternity patients. *Sociology of Health and Illness.* **15** (2): 157–78.

22   Ahmad WIU, Atkin K and Chamba R (2000) Causing havoc among their children: parental and professional perspectives on consanguinity and childhood disability. In: Ahmad WIU (ed) *Ethnicity, Disability and Chronic Illness.* Open University Press, Buckingham.

23   Kipple KF and King VIH (1981) *Another Dimension to the Black Diaspora.* Cambridge University Press, Cambridge.

24.   Rocherson Y (1988) The Asian mother and baby campaign: the construction of ethnic minority health needs. *Critical Social Policy.* **22**: 4–23.

25   Ahmad WIU (1993) *Race and Health in Contemporary Britain.* Open University Press, Buckingham.

26   Lipsky M (1980) *Street-Level Bureaucracy: dilemmas of the individual in public services.* Russell Sage Foundation, New York.

27   Darr A (1997) Consanguineous marriage and genetics: a model for genetic health service delivery. In: Clarke A and Parsons E (eds) *Culture, Kinship and Genes.* Macmillan Press, London.

28   Modell B and Darr A (2002) Genetic counselling and customary consanguineous marriage. *Nature Reviews Genetics.* **3**: 225–9.

29   Nazroo J (1997) *The Health of Britain's Ethnic Minorities.* Policy Studies Institute, London.

30   Mir G and Tovey P (In press.) Asian carers' experience of medical and social care: the case of cerebral palsy. *British Journal of Social Work.*

31   Green J and Statham H (1996) Psychological aspects of prenatal screening and diagnosis. In: Marteau T and Richards M (eds) *The Troubled Helix: social and psychological implications of the new human genetics.* Cambridge University Press, Cambridge.

32   Modood T, Betthould R, Lakey J *et al.* (1997) *Ethnic Minorities in Britain.* Social Policy Studies Institute, London.

33   Atkin K and Rollings J (1996) Looking after their own? Family caregiving in Asian and Afro-Caribbean communities. In: Ahmad WIU and Atkin K (eds) *Race and Community Care.* Open University Press, Buckingham.

34.   Ahmad WIU, Atkin K and Jones L (2002) Young Asian deaf people and their families: negotiating relationships and identities. *Social Science and Medicine.* **55** (10): 1757–69.

35   Hall S (1990) Cultural identity and diaspora. In: Rutherford J (ed) *Identity: culture, community and difference.* Lawrence and Wishart, London.

36   Husband C (1996) Defining and containing diversity: community, ethnicity and citizenship. In: Ahmad WIU and Atkin K (eds) *Race and Community Care.* Open University Press, Buckingham.

37   Chattoo S and Ahmad WIU (2003) The meaning of cancer: illness, biography and social identity. In: Kelleher D and Cahill G (eds) *Identity and Health.* Routledge, London.

38   Green J and Murton FE (1996) Diagnosis of Duchenne muscular dystrophy: parents' experiences and satisfaction. *Child Care, Health and Development.* **22** (2): 113–28.

39   Levick P (1992) The janus face nature of community care legislation: an opportunity for radical possibilities. *Critical Social Policy.* **12** (1): 75–92.

CHAPTER 3

Issues in the organisation and delivery of primary care

Philip Heywood

The previous chapter outlined the challenges facing primary care, as it struggles to provide accessible and appropriate provision. This chapter now refines our focus and specifically explores the organisation and delivery of primary care. My starting point, which further develops one of the implicit themes of the previous chapter, is that most users of the healthcare system have little choice but to accept what is offered to them and few are able to contribute to the design of the system before they use it. This is despite the fact that many who use the system and who are employed in the system, would prefer things to be different. This chapter is written from my personal and professional experiences as a white, Anglo-Saxon, male atheist. I will use those perspectives to consider how the current power structure in primary care has developed and suggest ways that may enable it to change to ensure better care for South Asian populations.

Defining primary care

It seems appropriate to start by defining what I mean by primary care and listing some of its key features. I use the term 'primary care' to mean those community-based health services that provide preventive, primary, personal and continuing care to patients and their families. There is an assumed responsibility for a population as well as for individuals. It is mainly a partnership between general practice and personal community health services, but includes the other contractor services (pharmacists, opticians and dentists) and some social services.[1]

Primary care has many features, which occur whatever the setting. The ideal service provides comprehensive care to the physical, psychological and social needs of individuals and their families. Comprehensive care includes health promotion and preventive care, first-contact healthcare, continuing care, rehabilitation and palliative care. It involves a direct therapeutic relationship between the patient/client and the professional. A team of clinical professionals supported by administrative staff deliver such care, all of whom engage in processes of continuing professional development. Primary care services are accessible and acceptable, and link appropriately to secondary healthcare and other health and social care agencies. It relates to the needs and to the resources of the community, and the community should be engaged in decisions about its care. It is underpinned by ongoing audit, evaluation and research.

How do these features of primary care relate to the explicit needs of minority ethnic communities? To fully explore this, every feature outlined above must be considered separately as each may have relevance for a patient, or for groups of patients, from South Asian populations.[2] South Asian patients, for example, may have specific physical, psychological and social needs; and these needs impact on health promotion and prevention as well as curative and supportive care. Continuing professional development programmes must include equal opportunities and anti-racist training as well as training that empowers practitioners to provide culturally sensitive services. Provision sometimes needs to be different to be acceptable and accessible. The responsiveness of services to minority communities must inform audit programmes, and research programmes must, in part, embrace minority issues.

This is what primary care should offer. In reality, medicine has a poor record of responding to the simplest needs of patients. In 1983, a survey by the Consumers' Association showed that 91 per cent of respondents wanted 'more time explaining about illness' from general practitioners (GPs) and 89 per cent wanted their GP to give 'more time listening to patients'.[3] Despite all the changes made to the NHS in the two decades since the survey, services have not changed in ways that responded to these wishes of patients. Indeed, there may be even less time for explanations and listening as the demands on GPs' time have become greater. This is particularly unfortunate as it may take more time to communicate effectively when a consultation occurs across linguistic and cultural barriers.

The creation of primary care trusts was supposed to offer an organisational mechanism for primary care to respond more appropriately to the needs of the community.[4] PCTs are responsible for defining the health needs of their population and they must then ensure that appropriate services are provided or commissioned to respond to those needs. As long as this definition of need is framed in ways that include South Asian populations' health needs, appropriate services can be provided. One mechanism that may help achieve this is the requirement to have representatives of the community on the board of the PCT. There has also been a belief over the last decade that people in primary care are nearer to patients than representatives of the former health authorities.[5] They are, therefore, thought to be better able to recognise those people's needs and ensure that services are appropriate: the rhetoric of a 'primary care-led NHS'.[6] It still remains to be proven whether or not this is the case.

If primary care is to provide new services, provide old services in new ways or commission different services from secondary care, it requires mechanisms for primary care development. Such developments should be driven towards a clear, coherent, achievable vision of future primary future: there must be a strategy to underpin each individual development and that strategy must have specific requirements for South Asian people. Further, primary care development must be founded on current practice and based on how it needs to change to achieve both its 'traditional' role and new or additional roles. It should be built on existing strengths and linked with other change mechanisms.

NHS commitment to equal opportunities

The NHS commitment to equal opportunities represents one of these change mechanisms. Three years ago it was stated that 'providing equitable healthcare to ethnic minorities is a key part of the NHS agenda'.[7] As the previous chapter demonstrated, however, it must be questioned whether this is any more than rhetoric. Perhaps, slowly, it is becoming a part of policy, but I will show that this is partial and explore some of the reasons why that may be so. Most people, whether users or providers, experience it, recognise it and know it to be the case. Nonetheless, because the NHS is in a state of flux, there is a possibility that ethnic sensitivity could become a real feature of future services offered within the NHS. Change does sometimes create the opportunity for radical possibilities.

In 2000, the Department of Health commissioned work by Ziggi Alexander to look at aspects of its work, including policy development, NHS and social care delivery, and workforce issues.[8] The following recommendations were made to equip staff in the health and social care services to meet the cultural, religious and language needs of local black and minority ethnic communities.

1   *Personal Development Plans for general practitioners and Practice Professional Development Plans for other practice staff will include a review mechanism to assess whether practices are meeting the needs of local patients, including black and minority ethnic communities.*
    This is admirable, but organisationally difficult to deliver. It assumes that such development plans are well developed in practices. They are not and, perhaps more importantly, they are most likely to be underdeveloped in the very practices that provide inappropriate services. These practices tend to be poor in many dimensions of their work; and the inverse care law highlights that poor practices often serve the most needy populations. Practitioners are required to find out from patients how they value a practice's services but they are not required specifically to enquire of their minority ethnic patients and there is little skilled help available to the average practice, for example, to develop appropriate instruments in minority languages or culturally sensitive approaches to consultation. A system of GP appraisal has only been introduced recently and already the specific issue of responding to minority ethnic communities has largely been lost.[9] All NHS employees need specific training in issues of race and racism, but such training is variable in its quality and in its effectiveness.
2   *National Service Frameworks will make explicit that the needs of black and minority ethnic communities must be addressed.*
    This is entirely reasonable, but there are problems practising evidence-based medicine when the research evidence is lacking. This is considered below under the theme of evidence-based healthcare.
3   *It is intended to establish a new project team to improve social care services for black and minority ethnic children and their families.*
    This has been slightly easier to implement as a new initiative, rather than the more difficult process of altering the behaviours of people in existing posts and existing organisations.
4   *NHS Direct, the nurse-led telephone advice line, must provide interpreting services and must respond to the specific needs of minority communities. It will be monitored for evidence of this.*
    One success over the last few years has been the increasing willingness of healthcare professionals to use telephone-based interpreting services. However, too many health professionals fail to recognise that they need to understand the patent's culture, as well as their language, if they are to respond

appropriately to a patient's needs. As we have seen in the previous chapter, providing appropriate language support is a far from straightforward matter.

5   *A clear understanding of the needs of minority ethnic communities will be built into all leadership and management development programmes.*

This is potentially an excellent way forward since such changes in organisations must be led from the top. The organisation will thrive if it regards its minority population as an opportunity to respond to its cultural diversity by being creative; it will, however, become defensive and embattled if it sees anti-racism as a series of pitfalls which it must avoid falling into.

6   *The pre- and post-registration training programmes of nurses and professionals allied to medicine must embrace issues of race.*

Many must have been surprised in 2000 to learn that training did not already embrace these issues. In 1995, the General Medical Council (GMC) published *Duties of a Doctor* that made explicit the high standards to which all doctors should aspire;[10] it is completely unacceptable for a doctor to discriminate on the grounds of race, ethnicity or religious beliefs. The then president of the GMC has described how professional self-regulation implies firstly a responsibility to the public (Irvine 1997).[11] All doctors have a duty to maintain good practice and patients must be protected from poor practice. The system will respond to racism, but the mechanisms for recognising such discriminatory behaviour are still poor.

Evidence-based healthcare in primary care

Many of Alexander's recommendations require the use of evidence-based healthcare and this is part of a much broader debate in healthcare. Evidence-based healthcare means the conscientious and judicious use of current best evidence from clinical care research in the management of individual patients. Perhaps it should always have happened. But it has not, sometimes for good reasons. The evidence base is generated by epidemiological study from populations of patients; it must then be applied to an individual. The evidence must be balanced by the doctor's clinical expertise and by the patient's preferences. The *evidence* says if a condition can be treated, whereas *clinical expertise*, in consultation with the patient, determines if it should be treated. But the weight of these three factors is unequal. Doctors sometimes fear evidence-based medicine because they believe it may subvert their experience as clinicians. It is, however, much more likely that the patient's perspective will be subverted, and this has particular implications for South Asian populations who already experience problems in gaining access to appropriate service delivery. There are also more specific difficulties in applying evidence-based healthcare in primary care. These problems relate to both the *research evidence* and *the setting of primary care*. Developing ideas explored in the previous chapter, this is a reminder that discrimination facing minority ethnic populations needs to be seen within the broader context of providing equitable primary care services for all.

Different forms of research evidence are accorded different value and there is an established hierarchy that judges the quality of evidence.[12] At the top of the hierarchy are high-quality systematic reviews and meta-analyses of randomised controlled trials (RCTs). One step lower lie RCTs, followed by non-randomised intervention studies. Next are observational studies, then non-experimental studies, and finally expert opinion. Randomised controlled trials require large numbers of research subjects and it is rare for there to be large numbers of people from minority populations in these trials. There are, therefore, few valid research results on which to base judgements.

Whenever data generated from populations are applied to an individual, it is necessary to judge the relevance of the data. For example, how well represented was *this* patient in the studies, particularly if the research subjects were drawn from a different ethnic group. There are many different outcomes of RCTs, such as speed of recovery; time to relapse; level of side effects; acceptability to patients; effect on usage of concurrent therapies. Which, if any, outcomes are paramount; and are they paramount for *this* patient? An RCT will not usually indicate the most cost-effective current treatment for general practice. Many interventions have been originally assessed within secondary care; how appropriate is that for subsequent application in primary care settings?

Treatments are usually administered to treat a specific patho-physiological diagnosis. Patients present in primary care with multiple and/or ill-defined problems, so it may be difficult to allocate a specific diagnosis to a symptom. Consultations may be triggered by a large number of circumstances (such as certification, external pressures, the need for social care), rather than a clinical event. Diagnoses and interventions are usually multiple, with physical, psychological and social elements. There are patients in whom the pathology is neither clear nor relevant to their problem, and even when there is pathology present, it is unusual in general practice for this to be confirmed by investigations. There may even be pressure to record a medical diagnosis to justify treatment.

Discrimination in primary care

Evidence-based medicine, as we have seen, raises generic issues for primary care and some of these issues might have particular implications for South Asian populations. I will now explore this further. Following publication of the Macpherson report, it has become clear that organisations may wield the power they have in ways that disadvantage groups of users (see also previous chapter). Unless active steps are taken to avoid discrimination, it will occur across a relationship where one party is disempowered. During my years in practice as a GP I have spent much of my time as a member of a minority community, a disempowered community, and followed that community in its journey to relative empowerment. That was within the community of general practitioners, who were weak compared to hospital consultants. The last decade has seen the power of GPs increase enormously relative to hospital doctors, first through GP fundholding and then through the establishment of PCTs. I fear that patients, however, may feel no difference unless professionals from primary care approach the exercise of power in different ways from those in the NHS who have previously held influence. I have no trite advice on how power can be wrested from professionals by service users and carers when primary care wields its influence inappropriately. Nonetheless, I shall consider those who work within the NHS who are from minority ethnic communities and who suffer the institutional racism, which is still present in the NHS, like many other British institutions.

Until the end of the last century, recruitment to medical school was racially biased.[13] Following McManus' publication, all medical schools have looked at their selection procedures and take great care to have non-discriminatory practices.[14] It is now less likely that there is racial discrimination in the selection of medical students. But there has long been discrimination in recruitment into various specialities, and into general practice training schemes. Racism has yet to be eliminated from primary care.[15,16] This racism is represented both in the acts and attitudes of individuals and in institutional racism. In his report into the death of Stephen Lawrence, Macpherson[17] defined institutional racism as 'the collective failure of an organisation to provide an appropriate service to people because of their colour, culture or ethnic origin'. In primary care this may affect any person from a minority ethnic background, whether user, carer, health professional or support staff.

Patterns of medical immigration between 1960 and 1980 mean that a large number of South Asian doctors came to the UK. Discriminatory promotion within the hospital system meant many Asian doctors failed to progress in hospital practice, and therefore sought careers in general practice. They now constitute a significant minority within primary care. Probably for reasons of discrimination, they are disproportionately represented in single-handed practices and in economically deprived areas. Although current policy is to reduce the number of single-handed practices there is no evidence that the care they provide is less good. Thus the desire to see larger practices flourish in preference to single-handed practices may, itself, be institutionally racist. Since that time there have also been increasingly large numbers of successful applications to medical schools by British Asian students. It is, therefore, likely that a significant proportion of GPs will continue to be of South Asian origin. Recruitment to nursing and professions allied to medicine differs slightly, but overall healthcare professions will continue to be a racially diverse group. It has been suggested that those who combine visible difference (for example, skin colour) with audible difference (for example, an accent) may be doubly disadvantaged.[18]

The extent to which Asian doctors experience racist abuse or actions from patients is not known. Anecdote suggests it is common; most ethnic minority doctors have experienced it. They have experienced proportionately more complaints from patients and the GMC, which investigates some complaints, has itself been judged possibly racist in its handling of ethnic minority doctors. Those who qualified outside the UK who are reported to the GMC are more likely than UK-qualified doctors to face the Professional Conduct Committee.[19]

The changing power of general practice and primary care

The care needs of South Asian populations, as we have seen, need to be debated in relation to the changing nature of primary care. This has been a central theme of this chapter and I would now like to specifically focus on the implications of altering power relationships within primary care for South Asian people. For the first eight decades of the last century, change came slowly to service organisation and delivery in general practice. Consequently, until the mid-eighties general practice had developed slowly. Prior to this, major organisational change had occurred every two decades, affecting most GPs only once or twice in their professional lives. The year 1911 saw the introduction of National Health Insurance for the working population; the GP's 'list' was born, initially insuring only the working population. A general practice service was thus created that was offered free at the point of access. Eighteen years later, in 1929, hospitals were moved into local authority control. Since many GPs held part-time hospital appointments, many of them lost their connection with secondary care. Nineteen years later, in 1948, the National Health Service was introduced, radically affecting the lives of GPs and severely affecting their quality of life through an initially unfair remuneration system. This unfairness led to increasing disenchantment, but was redressed 18 years later with the implementation of the Family Doctor's Charter in 1966. There were no further major organisational changes until 1990 when both a new charter, that rewrote the provision of primary care services, and *Working for Patients*,[5] that redefined primary care's relationship with secondary care, were introduced. Since then there has been no respite. The year 1996 provided legislation that allowed for pilot innovation to the provision of primary care services (PMS (personal medical services) pilots),[20] and in 1998 *The New NHS*[4] rapidly augmented these changes. Whereas general practice was previously a stable backwater of medicine, primary care is now in a constant state of change.

At the same time the position of general practice within the healthcare system has altered. As well as being geographically remote from the rest of medicine, it was organisationally remote. In the early 1950s, Lord Moran described how doctors arrived into general practice by falling off the ladder of promotion to consultancy.[21] They were in contract with organisations that were remote from power and decision taking, first the Executive Council, then the Family Practitioner Committee and finally the Family Health Services Authority. It was only in the 1990s that the GP's contract was finally held by the health authority, who was also contracted for hospital and community services.

GPs of different ages, as a group of citizens, bring very different experiences to their role. Those who are now entering practice, aged about 30 years old, grew up in Thatcher's Britain and trained wholly within the NHS after *Working for Patients* had been implemented. The remaining chapters contribute to these debates as they explore opportunities, grounded in the available evidence, to improve primary care outcomes for South Asian people. Thirty to 50-year-old GPs grew up in the welfare state, but they started to practise in the NHS prior to the changes of *Working for Patients*. Older GPs grew up before the state provided healthcare, and lived through the demoralisation of general practice in the 1960s. They saw many British-trained doctors emigrate and the NHS become dependent upon doctors trained abroad. It is therefore natural that these different groups of GPs see the current changes from different perspectives.

Group practice, compulsory vocational training for general practice, the Royal College of General Practitioners and university departments of general practice all contributed to the growth in stature, importance and power of the discipline. But the thing that really altered its position within the NHS organisation was fundholding.[5] This is particularly important because the most recent changes have merely amplified the power and influence that was initially bestowed on primary care by fundholding. *Working for Patients* introduced a system where the assessment of health needs and the commissioning of services became divorced from healthcare provision. Every institutional player was supposed to have the role of either a 'purchaser' or a 'provider'. The exception to this rule was general practice, which had a reciprocal relationship with every other player. For general medical services it was a provider to the health authority, but it partnered the health authority in its commissioning role and a few fundholding practices even supplied services, such as vasectomy or endoscopy, to the health authority. As purchasers, fundholding practices could obtain services from acute and community trusts as well as from private providers, but also from other fundholding practices. Finally, some practices worked with community trusts for the supply of community services.

The structure has, however, altered again. The basic block of *The New NHS* is the primary care trust. All the primary care providers for a defined population (usually between 50 and 150) are in a PCT. The PCT includes GPs and nurses as well as the other contractor professions, such as pharmacists, dentists and opticians. No primary care professional can opt out. A board leads the PCT and is supported by administrative staff.

Over the last 50 years clinicians had been almost entirely removed from NHS management. Although Sir Roy Griffiths bemoaned this in the mid 1980s,[22] the only move to redress it was the introduction of clinical directors in NHS trusts. Now, at a single stroke, clinicians are brought to the very centre of decision making about health. The PCT board includes about four doctors and nurses, although it has a majority of non-clinicians. In addition to the PCT board, which is responsible for the strategic direction of the PCT, there is also a Professional Executive Committee (PEC). The PEC is made up of clinicians from the area, and this group is responsible for delivering the board's strategy. It brings a large number of clinicians into the PCT management structure. PCTs are specifically charged with monitoring and improving the quality of services, in part through clinical governance. How optimistic can we be about the ability of boards to function well? The history of joint working between doctors and nurses in other than hierarchical relationships is not good. Further, GPs and social workers have also faced interprofessional relationship difficulties.

In summary, during a decade primary care has moved from the periphery of the health service to a central place. How likely are the practitioners to exercise their influence well, and to continue to devolve power further out? If they are like most other groups, not well. Having gained influence, and having realised that they have influence, they will try and keep it. Patients and users, who ultimately must take responsibility for their service, may have to fight the GPs for a greater say in how services are delivered.

The primary and secondary care interface

The final issue I wish to raise is the relationship between general practice and the secondary services. Firstly I shall consider why GPs make referrals, then something about the problem of shifting work from secondary to primary care. General practice has often been characterised as the gatekeeper to secondary care, but the role is seldom articulated. I believe there are seven conditions that must be met for a patient to avoid referral: hence every patient is a potential referral until the conditions are met:

1 Can an adequate level of diagnosis be achieved?
2 Can appropriate management/therapy be provided?
3 Is the prognosis better at home?
4 Have the carers the capacity to cope?

5 Has the patient the capacity to cope?
6 Are the home circumstances suitable?
7 Has the doctor the capacity to cope?
If yes to all of the above conditions, only then manage in primary care.

The reasons for referral listed above are not connected with the sort of pathol-ogy affecting the patient, or the nature of the patient, which are the two factors that underpin most referral protocols. The purpose underlying some of these protocols is to shift as much work as possible and appropriate from secondary to primary care. Overall it makes good sense to treat each patient in a setting that is as accessible, as economic and as comfortable as possible. Since, for many patients, a highly technical setting is uncomfortable, the familiar GP premises are prefer-able. Shifting work from primary to secondary care is fashionable, worldwide and politically motivated; it is partly a result of more high-tech interventions in second-ary care and reduction in the numbers of general specialists; it is perceived to be cheaper; however, it is not generally evidence based. Many of the people from primary care who negotiate such service shifts are experts in the field. Those who deliver it are GPs with no special expertise in the area. Although it is the least com-plicated hospital cases that are returned to general practice, they are, by definition, the most complex GP problems. We should therefore not be surprised at some resistance from primary care when we try to move services.

Conclusion

Just as we need to ensure that mainstream debates about ethnicity and health inform primary care development, we must also make sure that 'ethnicity and health' engages with what is going on in primary care. This and the previous chapter enable us to make this link, and by doing so provide a sustainable frame-work for making sense of ethnicity and primary care. The subsequent chapters develop this framework and provide more detailed insights that add support to primary care professionals in providing more equitable provision that is sensitive to the needs of South Asian people.

Returning to the core themes of this chapter, my first message was that primary care is in a state of flux and my second was that primary care clinicians are becoming central in decision making about healthcare. I asserted that the time is right for users to engage. This is especially true for minority ethnic users (as Chapters 4, 5 and 6 demonstrate). I predict that in those PCTs where the primary care clinicians are unchallenged, and where they are allowed to use their influence unbridled, services will be less responsive to patients than is those areas where there is real dialogue between users and providers. Timothy Milewa and Rukshana Kapasi provide good evidence of this in their chapter. Most PCT boards have difficulty knowing how to engage with users and carers and it is perhaps now timely for users and carers to identify themselves to their PCTs, to offer their perspectives, their experience and their commitment to their boards. In the absence of anything else, such approaches are likely to be embraced by many PCT boards and there is thus the opportunity for provision to be responsive to the needs of minority ethnic populations. As the previous chapter argued, disempowerment is not inevitable and minority ethnic communities have to engage in strategy and struggle to ensure their rights are recognised and met. If nothing else, the current state of flux informing primary care services creates opportunities for change.

References

1   Heywood P (2000) Primary health care: the changing character of service provision and use. In: Tovey P (ed) *Contemporary Primary Care and Change: issues and themes.* Open University Press, Buckingham.
2   Helman CG (2000) *Culture, Health and Illness.* Butterworth-Heinemann, Oxford.
3   Consumers' Association (1983) GPs. *Which?* **June**: 254–8.
4   Secretary of State for Health (1997) *The New NHS: modern, dependable.* Cmnd. 3087. Stationery Office Ltd, London.
5   Secretary of State for Health (1989) *Working for Patients.* Cmnd. 555. HMSO, London.
6   NHS Executive (1995) *Developing NHS Purchasing and GP Fundholding: towards a primary care-led NHS.* Department of Health, Leeds.
7   Department of Health (2002) *The NHS Plan.* HMSO, London.
8   Alexander Z (2000) *Study of Black, Asian and Ethnic Minority Issues.* Department of Health, London.
9   http://www.doh.gov.uk/gpappraisal
10 General Medical Council (1995) *Duties of a Doctor: good medical practice.* GMC, London.
11 Irvine D (1997) The performance of doctors. II. Maintaining good practice, protecting patients from poor performance. *BMJ.* **314**: 1613–15.
12 Harbour R and Miller J (2001) A new system for grading recommendations in evidence-based guidelines. *BMJ.* **323**: 334–6.
13 Abbasi K (1998) Is medical student selection discriminatory? *BMJ.* **317**: 1097–8.
14 McManus IC (1998) Factors affecting the likelihood of applicants being offered a place in medical schools in the UK in 1996 and 1997: retrospective study. *BMJ.* **317**: 1111–17.
15 Bhopal R (2001) Racism in medicine. The spectre must be exorcised. *BMJ.* **322**: 1503–4.
16 Coker N (ed) (2001) *Racism in Medicine. An agenda for change.* Kings Fund, London.
17 Macpherson W (1999) *The Stephen Lawrence Inquiry.* Stationery Office Ltd, London.
18 de Wildt G, Gill P, Chudley S *et al.* (2003) Racism and general practice – time to grasp the nettle. *British Journal of General Practice.* **53**: 180–2.
19 Dyer O (2003) GMC may be open to accusations of racial bias. *BMJ.* **326**: 411.
20 Lewis R and Gillam S (2002) Personal medical services. *BMJ.* **325**: 1126–7.
21 Irvine D (2001) The changing relationship between the public and the medical profession. *Journal of the Royal Society of Medicine.* **94**: 162–9.
22 Department of Health (1983) *NHS Management Inquiry (Griffiths Report).* HMSO, London.

PART 2

Meeting the needs of the service user

CHAPTER 4

Equity, clinical governance and primary care

Stephen Harrison

The main purposes of this chapter are to provide some conceptual clarity about notions of 'equity' in the context of healthcare, and to examine the concept of policy 'implementation' with special reference to new forms of primary medical care organisations in the English National Health Service. It gives specific expression to the broader issues raised in the previous chapter and will serve as background for subsequent chapters: both the substantive accounts of specific health problems and the discussions of how the NHS might contribute to greater equity for South Asian ethnic minorities. This conceptual background should make it clear that pursuit of such equity is far from unproblematic, for this is a subject matter where real discrimination and disadvantage meet genuine conceptual and organisational complexity and puzzlement. The following is divided into five sections. The first elucidates concepts of equity, highlighting those upon which NHS policies have tended to concentrate, showing that little systematic attempt has been made to address inequity for ethnic minorities. The second section examines the concept of implementation, whilst the third and fourth relate it to new organisational forms (primary care trusts) and processes (clinical governance) in NHS primary care. The final section concludes that, although the new National Service Frameworks may bring particular benefits to members of South Asian minorities, the requirements of clinical governance will in many cases inhibit any wider project of equity for them. Of course it does not follow from this that the project should be abandoned or attenuated and it seems possible that individual general practices, rather than the new larger primary care organisations, will be best placed to pursue it.

Conceptualising equity

The notion of equity implies both equal treatment for persons with equal needs, and a consistent relationship between the extent of their needs and the extent of their treatment. In order to employ this notion operationally, however, two of its dimensions must both be defined. First, we must define what is to count as 'treatment'; we might take this literally to mean actual healthcare interventions (often referred to in the literature as 'processes'), we might use money inputs as a proxy, or we might even look for equal health outcomes (which would strictly be *equality* rather than equity). Second, given that we cannot in practice examine whether every single individual has received what they need, we must decide what social groups are to be compared. Table 4.1 sets out as a matrix the broad choices provided by these requirements.

The horizontal axis of Table 4.1 represents what are perhaps the minimum possibilities for defining 'treatment': money inputs, processes and outcomes. Each of these could be further elaborated. The vertical axis contains some fairly obvious possibilities for social comparisons: class, age group, ethnic grouping, sex, sexual orientation, diagnostic category and geographically defined population. Again, this list is not exhaustive. It should be noted that of course these groups do not contain distinct groups of individuals. Rather, they are different ways of grouping those individuals and of potentially identifying the sources of their disadvantage, which may be multiple. For instance, individuals may suffer from the interaction between their ethnicity and their social class position (for a discussion of such 'difference within difference', see Harrison and Davis, 2001).[2] The consequences of this approach to defining equity are that each of the 21 cells in the matrix of Table 4.1 represents a possible definition. The operational definition of equity is thus not straightforward; if policy makers are to progress beyond rhetoric, they have to juggle a large number (21 on the above, relatively simplistic account) of options, not all of which they are likely to be able to pursue simultaneously.

It is not therefore surprising that, in practice, some cells seem of more concern to policy makers than do others. In the UK for instance, the NHS's resource allocation formula (a central policy concern for almost 30 years) is aimed at producing equity as defined in column 1 line 7 of the Table, though variables related to some of the other social groups are also included. At various times there has been concern in the UK about column 3 line 1 (health experience of different social classes, though the Black Report of 1980 was notoriously suppressed by the then government: Townsend and Davidson, 1983),[3] and about column 2 line 7 (differential geographic access to particular treatments, so-called 'postcode rationing'). There has been much less interest in line 3 (health and healthcare experience of different ethnic groups), despite the massive differences in such experiences which exist.

Table 4.1   Concepts of equity in health

	Inputs	*Processes*	*Outcomes*
Social class			
Age group			
Ethnic group			
Sex			
Sexual orientation			
Diagnostic category			
Geography			

Source: adapted from Harrison and Hunter (1994: p. 55)[1]

Conceptualising implementation

The world of public policy is one in which great emphasis is placed on policies, often at the expense of any concern with what happens afterwards. Put crudely, Ministers get their political credit for what they say they are going to do and for the institutions that they create to do it, rather than for the effects of their actions.

Box 4.1   The conditions for 'perfect implementation'

1   That there are sufficient material resources *in the appropriate combination* available to the programme. The question of resources thus goes beyond money; plentiful funds may not be able to overcome (say) skills or vaccine shortages and there must be no supply 'bottlenecks'.
2   That there are sufficient non-material resources (most obviously time and skills) available to the programme. Time is a non-trivial factor, since real-world organisations have ongoing activities and other priorities with which new policies have to compete for attention.
3   That the policy to be implemented is based upon a valid theory of cause and effect; it is only relatively recently that there has been a substantial discussion about 'evidence-based policy', and attempts to put it into practice are still rare.
4   That the relationship between cause and effect is direct and that there are few, if any, intervening links. The more links in the chain, the more likelihood that at least one will break down. If we see each link as an independent probability, the total probability of perfect implementation will be the product of all the individual probabilities; only ten links each with a (high) probability of 0.95 produces a total probability of 0.57, little better than evens!
5   That external dependency relations are minimal; this refers to political factors such as the refusal of other organisations to co-operate in implementing the policy. (The same mathematical considerations apply as in 4 above.)
6   Either
    • that internal dependency relations are minimal (this refers to internal organisational actors' propensity to obey instructions) *and* that the necessary tasks are fully specified in correct sequence (implying that policies should be capable of reduction to a detailed set of instructions). (The same mathematical considerations apply as in 4 above.)
    Or
    • that there is understanding of, and agreement on, objectives of the policy and how they are to be implemented, throughout the implementing organisation; that is, that there should be no conflicts within the implementing organisation and that everyone should clearly understand what they have to do and when.
7   That 'circumstances external to the implementing agency do not impose crippling constraints'. Such crippling circumstances might be natural factors such as epidemics or large-scale social factors such as economic crises.

As the NHS has become increasingly politicised over the last two decades, so the same kind of focus on the short term, on policies and on institutions has pervaded management. Gunn's (1978) notion of 'perfect implementation' provides us with some intellectual leverage on this trend by enabling us to identify the conditions that need to be considered if we are seriously concerned with implementation.[4] In my reformulation of Gunn's schema, there are seven conditions necessary for perfect implementation, set out in Box 4.1.

Of course, no one expects perfect implementation in the real world; the above approach describes a thought experiment as a means (as the case may be) of identifying the likely determinants of successful implementation, or of explaining unsuccessful implementation.

Clinical governance in the NHS

The New Labour government has officially defined 'clinical governance' as 'a framework through which NHS organisations are accountable for continuously improving the quality of their services and safeguarding high standards of care by creating an environment in which excellence in clinical care will flourish'.[5] In the official literature, the term is mainly used to refer to measures *within* NHS trusts, including PCTs. Such measures cannot, however, be understood other than in relation to the activities of new external institutions such as the National Institute for Clinical Excellence (NICE) and the Commission for Health Improvement (CHI). NICE has the role of undertaking evidence-based appraisals of new clinical interventions. Such appraisals may result in the production of 'clinical guidelines' for the management of relevant medical conditions, or in recommendations to the Department of Health that particular treatments should not be introduced to the NHS without further trials. Appraisals include evidence of *cost*-effectiveness as well as clinical effectiveness. National Service Frameworks, issued by the Department of Health, define the pathway through primary, secondary and tertiary care which a particular type of patient will be expected to pass and will be nationally promulgated, with compliance a dimension of NHS performance management. CHI will conduct a three- or four-year rolling programme of reviews, visiting every trust. Such reviews will include local compliance with clinical guidelines issued by NICE, and with NSFs. In addition to routine reviews, the Secretary of State, regional offices of the NHS Executive or health authorities will be able to initiate inquiries where local problems are suspected. Within trusts, the key element in the new arrangements is that chief executives are effectively responsible for the clinical, as well as the financial, performance of their institutions. New legislation places upon trusts a statutory duty for the quality of care. The activities of the new external institutions to which, given the new responsibilities of chief executives, there will presumably be a managerial motivation to respond, have clear implications for the *internal* control of provider institutions.

Clinical governance is thus a mechanism for controlling the health professions, most obviously doctors. The overall policy framework for steering the NHS is outlined in the document *A First Class Service: quality in the new NHS*.[5] Central to it is the application of a more rounded view of performance than adopted under the Conservative government; under the overall label of 'quality', this is outlined in the National Framework for Assessing Performance (NFAP)[6] as having six broad dimensions: health improvement, fair access, effective delivery of appropriate healthcare, efficiency, patient/carer experience and health outcomes of NHS care. Different dimensions of performance will be developed at a different pace. For example, within the third area ('effective delivery of appropriate healthcare'), three indicator sets are already the subject of consultation: clinical indicators, clinical effectiveness indicators and primary care effectiveness indicators. All NHS institutions will be subject to monitoring in terms of the extent to which quality of care and health have improved over time. The 'fair access' dimension of the NFAP described above corresponds to column 2 of Table 4.1, but most of the others can be construed as having equity aspects.

Clinical governance in NHS primary care

It is important to be neither excessively naïve nor excessively cynical about the ability of policy to impact on the pursuit of equity by organisations. Studies show that it can make a difference[7] but that it cannot be assumed to do so.[8] The advent of clinical governance provides a potential mechanism for the implementation of policies aimed at more equitable services. But in the context of PCTs, the probable efficacy of this mechanism is uncertain for two groups of reasons. First, they do not have a classical hierarchy, but rather are compulsory federations of small businesses, most often in the form of partnerships, though sometimes owned by a single practitioner. This is not to say that they do not have any of the features of hierarchy, but rather that the ownership structure of general medical practice attenuates their effect. The spread of salaried GP service to date does not yet suggest any rapid change in the ownership structure of general medical practice. Second, general practice seems to display a culture of independence which is consonant with the apparent lack of internal channels of authority: a general cynicism about government policy, a more specific perception that the latter need not really affect local matters, and the expectation of additional payment for any new task, suggesting that PCTs will have a limited capacity to implement bureaucratic rules and therefore to deliver the government's clinical governance agenda,[9] though there are perhaps some early indications of change (Harrison and Dowswell, forthcoming).

It is obvious that Gunn's conditions for perfect implementation are never likely to be fully met, even in the most authoritative top-down bureaucracy; it is even less likely that the kinds of primary care organisation that we have described above will manifest them. An exhaustive examination of the ten conditions is hardly necessary to show this. Consider, for instance: the importance of time (condition 2) in the context of GP work; the multi-agency effort which would need to be made in order to attack health inequalities (condition 5); conflicting policy priorities (condition 2) and the lack of unequivocal authority structures in primary care (condition 6). It is not surprising that primary care organisations are less likely than health authorities to address issues of ethnic inequality,[10] or that the former tend to express their priorities in terms of specific conditions such as coronary heart disease (Table 4.1, line 6) than to prioritise social groups.[11]

Concluding remarks

The analysis so far can be summarised in three statements. First, equity is a difficult and multifaceted concept to operationalise into clear objectives to which everyone in primary care could sign up. It implies giving a degree of priority to *particular* disadvantaged groups, an implication that at least some senior figures in the NHS find uncomfortable[12] and which might conflict with the current desperation to avoid 'postcode rationing'. Second, even if that were not so, the NFAP provides a wider range of other NHS performance targets, some of which compete with equity and others of which relate to equity in rather uncertain ways. In particular, concerns with equity conflict with dominant managerial notions of efficiency. The former have a primary concern with *distribution*; that is, they start from the position that there is a desirable allocation of whatever resources, services or outcomes are available, and aim to measure how far this has been achieved and/or to provide a guide as to how it can be achieved. In contrast, the latter starts from the assumption that outcomes across a society or population are to be *maximised*, and that the distribution of resources and services is secondary to this. Third, implementation is always likely to be difficult, but especially so in NHS primary care organisations. Finally, all these difficulties exist in a wider social context of racism in the UK.[13]

The content of political and policy agendas are rarely the result of a 'rational' search by policy makers of the many candidate issues. Studies show that the personification of issues through individual high-profile cases is one means by which they come to achieve genuine political salience.[14] Thus the issue of equity of higher educational opportunity has recently been embodied in the case of Laura Spence, a state school pupil rejected for the study of medicine at an élite university. The issue of racism generally is of course embodied in the case of the murdered black teenager Stephen Lawrence, but such personifications as have so far occurred in the field of healthcare equity have related either to 'postcode rationing' or to the disputed efficacy of new drugs. Even if issues attain the status of policy priorities, their translation into substantive action can easily become the casualty of competing demands for attention on the part of those organisational members whose role is to respond. Much effort in NHS primary healthcare is currently being devoted to the process of transition to new organisational forms and this may well be at the expense of attending to substantive health issues.[15] This potential priority overload is to some extent recognised in NHS performance management arrangements that allow local primary care organisations to choose many of their own clinical governance priorities, but it is not surprising that many have chosen the implementation of various NSFs as priority (Harrison and Dowswell, forthcoming) since they have to be implemented anyway. (It should be noted that some NSFs, most obviously those for coronary heart disease and diabetes, ought to offer particular benefits to members of South Asian ethnic minorities.) Whilst 16 per cent of a recent sample survey of primary care organisations report that they have identified ethnic minorities as having poor access to primary care,[16] it is not clear that this has so far resulted in any substantive action.

There are unlikely to be simple measures that will enhance the likelihood that NHS primary care organisations will be able to pursue greater equity for ethnic minority patients and communities. Much may depend on how the geographical concentration of South Asian populations differs in relation to particular primary care organisations. Where a PCT has a substantial ethnic minority population spread within its boundaries, it is feasible for equity of access to become a genuine clinical governance priority. PCTs tend, however, to be larger than their predecessors, implying that in most cases minority populations will be concentrated in specific parts of their territory. In such circumstances, it will be difficult to elevate ethnic minority healthcare to the highest level of clinical governance priority, implying that the pursuit of equity might fall to individual general practices.

Acknowledgements

Thanks are due to Waqar Ahmad and Sheila Paul for helpful comments on an earlier draft.

References

1   Harrison S and Hunter DJ (1994) *Rationing Health Care.* Institute for Public Policy Research, London.
2   Harrison ML and Davis C (2001) *Housing, Social Policy and Difference: disability, ethnicity, gender and housing.* Policy Press, Bristol.
3   Townsend P and Davidson N (1983) *Inequalities in Health: the Black Report.* Penguin, Harmondsworth.
4   Gunn LA (1978) Why is implementation so difficult? *Management Services in Government.* **33** (4): 169–76.
5   NHS Executive (1998) *A First Class Service: quality in the new NHS.* Department of Health, London.
6   NHS Executive (1998) *The New NHS: modern, dependable. A National Framework for Assessing Performance – a consultation document.* EL(98)4. Department of Health, London.
7   Thompson FJ (1981) *Health Policy and the Bureaucracy.* Massachusetts Institute of Technology Press, London.
8   Brewster CJ, Gill CG and Richbell S (1981) Developing an analytical approach to industrial relations policy. *Personnel Review.* **10** (2): 3–10.
9   Harrison S and Lim J (2000) Clinical governance and primary care in the English National Health Service: some issues of organisation and rules. *Critical Public Health.* **10** (3): 321–9.
10   Memon M, Abbas F, Singh I *et al.* (2001) Restricted access. *Health Service Journal.* **7 June**: 22–4.
11   Hayward J (1999) Thin on the ground. *Health Service Journal.* **26 August**: 26–7.
12   Foolchand M (2000) Behind closed doors. *Health Service Journal.* **13 April**: 32.
13   Ahmad WIU (ed) (1993) *'Race' and Health in Contemporary Britain.* Open University Press, Buckingham.
14   Solesbury W (1976) The environmental agenda: an illustration of how situations may become political issues and issues may demand responses from government, or how they may not. *Public Administration.* **54** (4): 379–97.
15   Wilkin D, Gillam S and Smith K (2001) Primary care groups: tackling organisational change in the NHS. *BMJ.* **322**: 1464–7.
16   Abbott S and Gillam S (2001) Health Improvement. In: Wilkin D, Gillam S and Coleman A (eds) *The National Tracker Survey of Primary Care Groups and Trusts 2000/2001: modernising the NHS?* University of Manchester National Primary Care Research and Development Centre, Manchester.

CHAPTER 5

User involvement in primary healthcare: problems, paradigms and prospects

Timothy Milewa and Rukshana Kapasi

This chapter examines public and patient involvement in primary healthcare with particular regard to people of South Asian origin or descent. The previous chapter examined clinical governance and implied that challenging health inequalities is far from straightforward and requires collective action. This chapter begins to explore the implications of this further, by exploring the extent to which user involvement influences primary healthcare. The chapter is in five parts. We first outline recent policy interventions with regard to involvement. The second part of the chapter then considers reasons why service planners and providers should pay particular attention to South Asian minority ethnic populations when designing and conducting initiatives in involvement. In section three we focus upon involvement in strategic context by considering some of the main rationales and assumptions that shape the purpose, intended outcome and impact of public and patient involvement. We then provide some specific examples of early attempts to engage minority ethnic groups by relatively new organisations in the health service: primary care groups (PCGs) and primary care trusts. The final part of the chapter considers some of the main issues to be borne in mind by planners and providers in the development of involvement strategies and initiatives that are more sensitive to the needs of minority ethnic groups.

Policy context

Public and patient involvement in the planning and delivery of healthcare has been a recurrent feature of government policy and exhortation since the early 1990s. The division between health service commissioners and providers was accompanied by an official depiction of local people as 'advisors' to health authorities in the commissioning and development of local health services. One much-cited advisory document, *Local Voices*, listed mechanisms by which to gauge the opinions of local populations and particular service user groups: these included community forums, postal questionnaires, focus groups and other means.[1] The importance attached by the government to the *Local Voices* initiative varied between 1992 and 1997, but the impact of public and patient involvement activities on decision-making processes in the health service was, at best, varied.[2–4] Subsequent movement towards a 'primary care-led' health service has also been accompanied by an emphasis on enhancing the 'local responsiveness' of services through the use of public and patient involvement mechanisms.

The foundation in England of 481 groups of local GPs and other primary care professionals – called primary care groups in their non-statutory stage and primary care trusts upon achieving autonomous legal status – centred on the delivery and commissioning of primary care and some aspects of secondary care.[5] The PCGs/PCTs were also expected by the Department of Health to develop mechanisms for the 'early, systematic and continuous involvement of users and the public'.[6] These mechanisms and processes will, the government claims, help PCTs to 'work with their local communities to develop shared goals and aims for improving local health and well-being'. Accordingly, 'patient and public involvement needs to be integral to the way in which PCGs work'.[7] More specifically, for the purposes of this chapter, the Race Relations (Amendment) Act 2000 imposes upon all public authorities, including PCTs, several duties of direct relevance to the involvement of people from minority ethnic groups. Public bodies must, wherever relevant, consult minority ethnic representatives; take account of the potential impact of policies on minority ethnic groups; monitor the impact of policies and services with regard to different ethnic groups and, in a fourth regard, take remedial action when necessary to address unexpected or unwarranted disparities.

Primary healthcare providers and planners in areas within which minority ethnic groups form a significant part of the population are therefore obliged to consider particular involvement strategies and mechanisms for these citizens and service users. But are there any other reasons, beyond government edicts, for addressing the concerns of people from minority ethnic groups in general and people of South Asian origin or descent in particular?

Why focus on involving minority ethnic groups?

Most obviously, different parts of the population can and do differ significantly with regard to particular health problems and healthcare needs. We know, for example, that the prevalence of diabetes is much higher among people of South Asian origin or descent living in England than in the population as a whole. The prevalence of diabetes among Indian men is almost three times that of the male general population while the prevalence among Pakistani and Bangladeshi men is over five times that of men as a whole: marked disparities are also evident among women from these backgrounds. Indian, Pakistani and Bangladeshi men also have a higher prevalence of ischaemic heart disease and angina than the general male population. In terms of perceptions, the prevalence of long-standing illness that sufferers say interferes with their normal activities is much higher among men and women of Pakistani and Bangladeshi origin/descent than among other ethnic groups. Indeed, when people were asked to assess their general health, Bangladeshi men and women were over three times more likely to use the descriptions of 'bad' or 'very bad' than the male or female populations in general – a marked tendency also evident among men and women of Indian or Pakistani origin or descent. Similarly, with regard to perceived physical and emotional support from family and friends, men and women from all three of these groups were over twice as likely as the wider male and female populations to report a lack of such support.[8]

It is, however, important in the development of involvement initiatives that such statistics are only used as *background* to consideration of how the needs and preferences of minority ethnic populations might be gauged. We know, for example, that household income has been shown to have a relationship with the predisposition of men of Indian or Pakistani origin/descent to report long-standing illness that limits everyday activities. Those in the lowest income bracket are more likely than the male population as a whole to report such limiting illness but those in the highest income bracket are less likely to make such a claim than the male population in general. In more concrete terms, the danger of treating particular minority ethnic groups as coherent entities for the purposes of planning was also illustrated by a localised survey of Asian older people's use of GP services. The results suggest that 81 per cent of informants thought that contacting and consulting their GPs was relatively easy. But, again, closer examination of the statistics shows that only 63 per cent of Asian women in the sample felt that this was the case.[9] Indeed, black and minority ethnic communities are generally much more reluctant to complain about poor services than other population groups, despite the fact that they often have substantial concerns about the accessibility, quality and appropriateness of the services they receive.[10]

Challenging assumptions on the part of healthcare providers

Simply focusing on the attitudes and preferences of ethnic minority patients overlooks another potential obstacle to their expression of needs and preferences: the values and behaviour of healthcare practitioners and managers themselves. At a general level, engaging individuals and families from ethnic minority backgrounds through mechanisms for public and patient involvement is one way to challenge a priori ideas held by some healthcare providers about ethnic minority cultures. Such assumptions may not only compound existing difficulties based on language,[11] but also influence the quality of healthcare provided – an influence that manifests itself at three levels.

At one level, professional assumptions about minority ethnic groups may generate and perpetuate racial stereotypes, such as the association drawn by some white midwives in one study between prolonged silence on the part of Asian clients and 'stupidity'. Similarly, the failure by some Asian clients to use 'please' or 'thank you' in verbal exchanges was interpreted by some practitioners as rudeness, with little allowance made for the clients' lesser knowledge of verbal cues and idioms in the English language. And at a second level, such perceptions do not simply detract from mutual respect and effective communication but can have a demonstrable impact on service provision. Research has suggested, for example, that medical professionals are sometimes reluctant to test South Asian prospective parents for thalassaemia on the grounds that people from this 'culture' tend not to contemplate terminations of pregnancy or on the basis that positive results would be of little use in influencing family decisions to terminate.[12] Indeed, in a third regard, this 'racialised' framing of issues can influence the very existence or development of health services of particular relevance to minority ethnic populations.[13] A failure to acknowledge the multi-ethnic nature of society can, in effect, slow down the development of appropriate services.[14]

Clearly, a 'statistical' awareness of the healthcare needs of minority ethnic populations has to be accompanied by an acknowledgement of the need to avoid or challenge preconceptions and stereotypes when developing involvement or consultation initiatives. But, even assuming that such an awareness exists on the part of primary healthcare planners and providers, 'involvement' itself is far from straightforward. Most obviously, there is the issue of what health service planners and providers want from involvement.

What is involvement for?

The mechanisms of involvement are, in one way, quite straightforward. Various official and semi-official guides, such as the *Reference Manual for Public Involvement*, *The Public Engagement Toolkit* and *Listen Up!*, have been circulated widely – these offer advice, for example, on the design of questionnaires, the conduct of focus groups, interactive media and systems for feeding back information to the public and patients.[15–17] The type of involvement mechanism chosen and the reasons for choosing it can have radically different implications for both the involved and those doing the involving. Harrison (1999), for example, suggests that there are four major types of public and patient involvement (*see* Box 5.1)[18]

Any of the four types of involvement will, however, be restricted in their impact if the broader purpose of gauging public and patient views is unclear to service planners. As already noted, primary healthcare planners and providers have been under sustained pressure to demonstrate activity around public and patient involvement, but considerably less emphasis has been placed on proving associated outcomes. Involvement may thus, in some circumstances, be essentially 'ceremonial' or token in nature.[19] So, despite being described as participants, patients and members of the public may remain observers without real access to decision making. There is thus the risk that professionals will subscribe to the rhetoric of involvement but do

---

Box 5.1   Types of public and patient involvement

1   *Deliberated and informed involvement* whereby those whose views are being sought are provided with fairly detailed background information by service planners or providers. The participants then reflect at length on the material in a way that they deem fit before reaching their own conclusions or recommendations (e.g. citizens' juries).

2   *Deliberated and uninformed involvement* where participants consider issues but are not provided with significant background information and may often be guided by facilitators (e.g. some focus groups, discussion groups).

3   *Undeliberated and informed involvement* where those whose views are being sought are given some background information but their answers largely reflect a predetermined set of options (e.g. 'closed-response' questionnaires that are supplemented by explanatory information).

4   *Undeliberated and uninformed involvement* reflects exercises in which respondents are given no background information while the list of possible answers is largely predetermined (e.g. *ad hoc* fixed-response questionnaires to randomly selected samples of the population).

no more than manipulate the process to legitimise their own decisions and inter-ests.[20,21] Alternatively, attempts to involve people from minority ethnic groups may, for example, be premised on a perceived need to make them aware of local services that they appear to underutilise or to discourage a perceived overutilisation of certain services. In a third regard, involvement may simply reflect attempts to ensure that voices not normally heard are given the chance to contribute to relevant debates in ways that more 'mainstream' sections of society have participated: an 'equal opportunities' approach to involvement. This approach might typically centre upon the provision of written information in minority ethnic languages, the employ-ment of bilingual staff and the provision of professional translators in the course of medical consultations.[22] But a fourth approach may be specifically 'anti-racist' in that it is premised on a view that minority ethnic groups' experience of healthcare provision is often influenced by discriminatory attitudes and behaviours on the part of service planners and providers. Mechanisms such as focus groups, regular forums and advisory committees will thus concentrate not only on the technical aspects of service planning but also seek to challenge and confront attitudes that are seen to be racist.[23]   Finally, in a fifth respect, the involvement of minority ethnic groups may sit within wider strategies designed to alleviate health inequalities, combat deprivation and empower all sections of the community to participate in a broad range of relevant debates: a 'community development' approach.[24]

This last point illustrates perhaps the most fundamental issue with regard to involvement activities: whose agenda is being addressed and who decides what are legitimate topics for debate? Clearly, involvement in health service planning entails a focus on local health services and related provision, perhaps in the social care field. But it is important to distinguish between debates instigated and imposed by plan-ners and providers and those topics considered important by local communities and patients. In this last respect, planners in the health service should keep in mind groups whose priorities and assumptions reflect an organisational autonomy and strategic self-determination on the part of participants. Begum *et al.* (1994), for example, report on some self-organising aspects of the black disabled people's movement,[25] while Ahmad *et al.* (1998) focus on the processes whereby minority ethnic deaf people are self-organising not only around a 'deaf identity' but also with regard to ethnic and religious symbols.[26]

Clearly, different stakeholders may perceive involvement in terms of radically different motives and objectives – factors that are central both to the design and evaluation of subsequent initiatives. But, more immediately, is there any indication that the relatively new primary healthcare organisations mentioned earlier, PCGs and PCTs, are at least beginning to give some thought to gauging the views of minority ethnic groups?

What kind of involvement is going on?

The issue of minority ethnic involvement formed part of a survey of PCGs and PCTs in late 1999 and early 2000.[27] A random sample of chief executives of half the groups outside London were asked to nominate spokespersons for tele-phone interviews: 167 interviews were conducted (a response rate of 80 per cent). Sixty-seven of the PCG/PCTs (40 per cent) indicated that some of their public and patient involvement activities had been aimed specifically at what they regarded as 'marginalised' groups. These informants were then asked, *without prompting*, to identify the marginalised groups they had in mind. The responses were obviously influenced by local conditions and agendas but, overall, minority ethnic communities were cited more frequently than any other groups, accounting for 26 per cent or 29 of the 111 nominations. In comparative terms, older people and 'deprived' communities accounted for about 16 per cent of nominations each and mentally ill people for just over 15 per cent. Other groups identified included the physically disabled (7 per cent) and people with learning difficulties (4.5 per cent). More specifically, 25 of the 29 informants who had identified minority ethnic groups as 'marginalised' claimed to be developing or implementing related involvement activities and were able to cite 55 specific initiatives.

These activities fell into several distinct categories. The largest cluster, accounting for 17 of the 55 examples (31 per cent), reflected meetings between PCG/PCT directors and managers and ethnically based voluntary, community or patient groups. These included, for example, meetings held at Bangladeshi and Pakistani community centres and with a Black and Asian women's group. Three other categories of involvement accounted for 11 per cent each of the activities mentioned. First, specially convened, one-off public meetings focused on issues that included the development of diabetic services with particular regard to Asian service users while another meeting discussed minority ethnic issues in the development of a local health improvement plan. In a second respect, some activities centred on written or electronic media. Examples included a series of radio programmes on health issues in minority ethnic languages that were followed by workshops and an 'IT Health Day' that sought to demonstrate how health advice could be accessed by people from minority ethnic groups. In another category, a similar proportion of activities centred on PCG/PCT representation on existing, independent networks – these included an Asian health and social care forum. Other categories of involvement activities included meetings with 'opinion leaders' (9 per cent), questionnaires (7.3 per cent) and interview-based surveys (3.6 per cent).

This snapshot of involvement activities demonstrates at least some consideration on the part of primary healthcare managers and providers of issues pertaining to minority ethnic groups. But the survey came at a very early stage in the development of PCG/PCTs and the British health service remains, of course, open to continuing reform. So are there more general, omnipresent principles around the involvement of minority ethnic groups?

South Asian populations and involvement: issues in strategy and implementation

We end this chapter by exploring the strategic and operational considerations and principles to be kept in mind when involving minority ethnic populations in primary healthcare. We begin by exploring the strategic implications. Public and patient involvement, together with appreciation of the needs of groups that are perceived to be marginalised, are ideas to which any organisation can subscribe. But ensuring that the principles are ensconced in practice depends upon at least five factors.

First, it is important that in the context of a national but locally diverse health service there remains sustained pressure, encouragement and monitoring from the government or its agencies with regard to public and patient involvement. This need was illustrated, for example, in plans for all NHS trusts to have in place patient advisory services (PALS) by early 2002.[28] The first review of PALS pilot sites indicated that very few PALS had considered diversity as an integral part of their structures.[29] Secondly, in more operational terms, the impact of public and involvement activities is highly dependent upon assumptions about the purpose of involvement, the intended participants and the use to which feedback will be put. Clarifying and enunciating these assumptions is therefore essential at the outset. In a third, related regard, effective involvement of minority ethnic groups will often depend upon preliminary discussion with such constituents about the health and healthcare issues that they feel are important, the means by which they would prefer to be involved and clear specification of what will happen to opinions that emerge. In a fourth respect, an inclusive approach to involvement will hinge upon a managerial/professional enthusiasm that is consciously suffused throughout service planning and delivery organisations. Mechanisms and strategies might include internal newsletters, staff workshops and participation by personnel at all levels in events designed to engage the public and patients.[30] Indeed, awareness of minority ethnic health needs and problems might also form a part of management training and development courses and feature on the curricula of undergraduate healthcare courses in fields such as general practice and nursing. Finally, professional awareness and commitment will only be sustained if it is reflected in explicit, written, organisational standards and expectations around involvement, clear mechanisms of accountability for the observance of such standards and effective systems for monitoring and review.[31] Indeed, where bodies such as PCG/PCTs are in a position to enter into contractual arrangements with service providers – such as general practices or hospitals – stipulations concerning involvement and consultation may also be included in contracts concerned with service delivery and associated procedures.

We now turn to the process of implementation and at a practical level a number of basic measures will improve accessibility to consultation and involvement. Perhaps most obviously, given the ongoing nature of attempts to engage the public and patients within the NHS, PCTs need to invest time in groundwork with local minority ethnic communities to convince them that they are serious and genuinely interested in listening to and acting upon local views. Many communities may have 'clipboard fatigue' from previous involvement initiatives that have yielded little demonstrable change.[32] Other measures include:

- provision of language interpreters to facilitate communication with non-English speaking groups
- use of bilingual advocates or existing minority ethnic community workers to explain the purpose of consultation and explain the new primary care structures and systems
- publicity in appropriate languages with imagery that is 'inclusive'
- reimbursement of travel expenses or provision of transport to accessible and familiar community venues
- availability and choice of a range of methods of involvement to take account of single sex preferences and the fact that many isolated communities may not feel comfortable in expressing themselves at large group events

- working with and building on the work of existing community networks, groups and organisations who have established a positive relationship with a range of communities.

The degree to which planners, practitioners and of course minority ethnic groups can realise these principles will be central to determining whether 'involvement' is based on more than just rhetoric for minority ethnic groups such as South Asian populations.

References

1   NHS Management Executive (1992) *Local Voices: the views of local people in purchasing for health*. National Health Service Management Executive, London.
2   Pickard S (1998) Citizenship and consumerism in healthcare: a critique of citizens' juries. *Social Policy and Administration*. **32**: 226–44.
3   Mort M, Harrison S and Dowswell T (1999) Public health panels in the UK: influence at the margins. In Khan UA (ed) *Innovations in Political Participation*. Taylor and Francis, London.
4   Association of Community Health Councils for England and Wales (1999) *Commission on Representing the Public Interest in the Health Service*. Association of Community Health Councils for England and Wales, London.
5   Wilkin D, Gillam S and Leese B (2000) *The National Tracker Survey of Primary Care Groups and Trusts: progress and challenges 1999/2000*. University of Manchester National Primary Care Research and Development Centre, Manchester.
6   Department of Health (1998) *Developing Primary Care Groups*. LAC(98)21. Department of Health, London.
7   Department of Health (1999) *Patient and Public Involvement in the New NHS*. Department of Health, London.
8   Department of Health (1999) *Health Survey for England: the health of minority ethnic groups, 1999*. Department of Health, London.
9   Ahmad WIU and Walker R (1997) *Asian Older People: housing, health and access to services*. (Report.) Department of Social and Economic Studies, University of Bradford, Bradford.
10 Association of London Government (2000) *Sick of Being Excluded: improving the health of London's black and minority ethnic communities*. Association of London Government, London.
11 Vydelingum V (2000) South Asian patients' lived experience of acute care in an English hospital. *Journal of Advanced Nursing*. **32** (1): 100–7.
12 Atkin K, Ahmad WIU and Anionwu EN (1998) Screening and counselling for sickle cell disorders and thalassaemia, *Social Science and Medicine*. **47** (11): 1639–51.
13 Ahmad WIU (ed) (1993) *'Race' and Health in Contemporary Britain*. Open University Press, Buckingham.
14 Tovey P, Atkin K and Milewa T (2001) The individual and primary care: service user, reflexive choice maker and collective actor. *Critical Public Health*. **11** (2): 153–66.

15 Barker J, Bullen M and de Ville J (1997) *Reference Manual for Public Involvement.* NHS South Thames, London.

16 NHS Executive Northern and Yorkshire (1999) *Public Engagement Toolkit.* NHS Executive Northern and Yorkshire, Durham.

17 Audit Commission (1999) *Listen Up! Effective community consultation.* Audit Commission, London.

18 Harrison S (1999) *Innovations in Citizen Participation in Government: a note on citizen participation in the NHS for the Select Committee on Public Administration, 1999–2000.* (Document.) Nuffield Institute for Health, Leeds.

19 Richardson A (1983) *Participation.* Routledge and Kegan Paul, London.

20 Brownlea A (1987) Participation: myths, realities and prognosis. *Social Science and Medicine.* **25** (6): 605–14.

21 Harrison S and Mort M (1998) Which champions, which people? Public and user involvement in health care as a technology of legitimation. *Social Policy and Administration.* **32** (1): 60–70.

22 Shah A and Piraka A (1993) *Hello, Can You Hear Me? A study of the communication experiences of the Asian community with health services in Blackburn, Hyndburn and Ribble Valley Health Authority.* Blackburn, Hyndburn and Ribble Valley Health Authority, Blackburn.

23 Wilson R, Tate S and Boughan S (2000) *Committing to Equality: community health councils in the Northern and Yorkshire Region.* Regional Association of Community Health Councils, Northern and Yorkshire, Leeds.

24 Bradford City Council (2000) *Building Communities: the five-year strategy and action plan on community development for the district of Bradford.* (Document.) Bradford City Council, Bradford.

25 Begum N, Hill M and Vernon A (1994) *Reflections: the views of black disabled people on their lives and community care.* Central Council for Education and Training in Social Work, London.

26 Ahmad WIU, Darr A, Jones L *et al.* (1998) *Deafness and Ethnicity: services, policy and politics.* Policy Press, Bristol.

27 Milewa T, Harrison S, Ahmad W *et al.* (2002) Citizens' participation in primary health care planning: innovative citizenship practice in empirical perspective. *Critical Public Health.* **12** (1).

28 Department of Health (2001) *Involving Patients and the Public in Healthcare: a discussion document.* Department of Health, London.

29 Kapasi R and Silvera S (2001) *A review of the London PALS pathfinder sites.* London Regional Office, London.

30 Milewa T and Calnan M (2000) Primary care and public involvement: achieving a balanced partnership. *Journal of the Royal Society of Medicine.* **93** (1): 3–5.

31 Silvera M and Kapasi R (2001) *Health Advocacy for Black and Minority Ethnic Londoners.* King's Fund, London.

32 Alves B, Kapasi R, Silvera M *et al.* (2000) *An Evaluation of the Primary Care Ethnicity Project.* London Regional Office, London.

CHAPTER 6

Better partnerships, better services

Dee Kyle

This chapter, which concludes Part 2 of the book, offers a more pragmatic response to achieving equity in primary healthcare by focusing on a specific service example. To this extent, it is very different from the other chapters in this volume and offers a personal reflection on the dilemmas faced by health professionals as they struggle to deliver better services to South Asian populations. My particular concern is with how building better partnerships can improve health services for South Asian communities. I begin my account by reflecting on the reasons for improving service support for South Asian people. I then go on to describe some of the key principles and requirements in building partnerships, by presenting examples, grounded in the realities of service delivery, of successful outcomes.

Improving primary health care for South Asian populations: the need for empathy, curiosity and respect

Several reasoned arguments can be put forward for the need to improve health services for South Asian populations communities. First, as we have seen in previous chapters, the NHS like many organisations has struggled with racism, institutional racism and ethnocentricity. Second, we have recently rediscovered that health outcomes are not just influenced by the availability of services to diagnose and treat disease. Prevention is equally important. In 1974, the preventive health services of the local authority were integrated into the NHS and the Royal College of General Practitioners increasingly supported a shift of practice in primary care towards prevention and health promotion as well as diagnosis and treatment. Public health specialists aim to improve the health of the public through programmes that protect health and improve health as well as those which improve the effectiveness and efficiency of health services. Increasingly, services are being planned, delivered and monitored in direct response to health needs. This requires the NHS, patients and public to have a greater understanding of the health needs of different communities, such as South Asian populations, for both prevention and treatment, as well as an awareness of the need for the involvement of others outside the NHS. Thirdly, the availability of health services does not guarantee their accessibility, acceptability and appropriateness. Effective communication between service users and providers is essential if services are to become accessible, acceptable and appropriate. This includes overcoming language difficulties not only to ensure basic comprehension between patients and professionals, but also to promote understanding and information about health, health needs and how they can be met. As we have seen in previous chapters, cultural differences can affect accessibility, acceptability and appropriateness of primary healthcare services.

As part of this, communication skills are also increasingly recognised as basic components of the education of health professionals. In the USA, culturally competent communication skills are becoming part of both basic training and continuing professional development. Carrillo et al. (1999)[1] describe a curriculum to deliver such skills based on a model of empathy, curiosity and respect. They point out that this is what 'good doctoring' is all about: listening, asking the right questions and meeting the patients' needs. In the context of primary care this means finding out about the ideas, concerns and expectations of patients and negotiating appropriate action. To do this across cultural differences and language barriers takes more time and needs additional skills. The principles of empathy, curiosity and respect need to permeate all levels of service planning and provision and not just individual patient consultations. In the UK until very recently, the principle of provision of 'comprehensive services free at the point of use' has allowed the responsibility for cross-cultural communication to rest squarely with potential users: 'come and get it' – but on 'our' (the powerful majority) terms (see also Chapter 2).

Research on the health needs of South Asian communities, as previous chapters demonstrate, have at best been inadequate and at worst compounded discrimination. Inadequate because South Asian populations have frequently been explicitly excluded on the grounds that there is no time to explore issues if potential patients are not fluent in English; or that standardised research tools (such as questionnaires and measurement scales) have not been validated on these populations. Discriminatory because of ethnocentric selectivity as to what is researched ('interesting' if rare, single gene conditions) or how it is researched – assumptions leading to unhelpful labelling, classification or stereotyping.

An inadequate knowledge of needs and poor levels of competency in cross-cultural communication can lead to the conclusion that poor health outcomes in South Asian populations are at least in part the result of inaccessible, unacceptable and inappropriate health services (see Chapter 2). There are ways to reverse this trend and improve services for South Asian communities by building partnerships. I will now explore key features of building partnerships and give examples of successful outcomes when working at a local level.

Partnerships: the key to improving services for South Asian populations

When discussing partnership, three factors are particularly important. First, culturally competent communication is necessary but that alone is not sufficient to improve the outcome of services. To overcome the barrier of communication is one thing; equally important is the content of the communication. Good communication requires empathy (the ability to imagine oneself 'in the other person's shoes'), curiosity (interest in the person with whom one is communicating) and a respect for their point of view. To this extent, the individual needs to be helped to access services which are empathic (provided in ways which make them feel that their needs are understood), curious (about their needs) and respectful (of their cultural and religious background and sensitivities). Requests made for circumcision for cultural or religious reasons offer an example of this.

Secondly, a realistic partnership between providers and users of services is essential for good health outcomes (see Chapter 5). Service users are no longer prepared to allow health professionals to make all the decisions for them and wish to have more of a say in the services provided for them. Even if people are prepared to trust totally the professionals and 'obey' their instructions, the active participation of service users is also required. This is especially important for prevention, and for chronic disease management – where the 'expert patient' concept is developing, building on the experience gained from living with their condition – and for promoting 'concordance' on ever more complicated treatment regimens.

Thirdly, not all services that improve health are 'health services'. Children, for example, with diabetes reported that they felt a key component of their health and well-being was their school's understanding of their condition. Multifaceted partnerships between health services, patients and families, and others that have the power to improve health are increasingly being accepted as necessary for health gain. As *The NHS Plan* proposes, the roles of primary care professionals are changing from being seen as 'gatekeepers' to health services to being 'signposters' and 'providers' of a wide range of services essential for good health (such as advice on social security benefits, social care, housing and employment).[2]

Key principles and requirements for partnership working

At a strategic level, a partnership needs to be formed between community representatives (service users), front-line workers and managers who have influence in service planning and delivery. The partnership needs to be action-oriented by ensuring that the information generated out of the empathy, curiosity and respect of the partnership is tightly linked to strategic decision making to allow the user perspective to feed into the process of service development. In this way issues which users perceive as priorities requiring action can be highlighted and translated into action by service planners and be promoted through the joint planning processes in general and modernisation processes in PCTs.

An important level of partnership is the provision of health services by members of the community, in the community's first languages. The provision of mental health services for South Asian women by South Asian women in the users' first language has begun to build the partnerships required to improve mental health services for South Asian populations in Bradford. This was largely a response by service providers to the experiences of some South Asian populations users who described their admission to mental health inpatient facilities as if they had been 'abducted by aliens'. Service names in Asian languages, such as 'Roshni Ghar' ('House of Light'), 'Naya Subha' (New Dawn) and Jyoti (Light), have helped South Asian communities to relate to NHS services better and are better appreciated by users. Partnerships are also being forged with 'harder to reach' groups, such as young people who, in all cultures, see less need for 'health services', especially those provided by and oriented towards adults. An example of this is 'No to Nasha' ('No to intoxication') which tackles the need to engage on sensitive subjects, including illegal drug use, on the terms and with the involvement of the young people themselves. It uses drama and music (such as 'bangrah') to engage the interest of young people and through drama allows the expression of intergenerational tensions and issues in a humorous and non-threatening way.

Most older South Asian people tend to converse mainly in Urdu, but for younger South Asian people, it is usually English. Designing projects with the capacity to work in both languages has enabled partnership between generations to be established around health issues. For example, a local Youth Partnership Project linked the younger and older generations of South Asian populations in discussing health issues. Most of the work was performed in South Asian populations' languages, and older women were keen to be involved in discussing health issues and helped highlight problems areas whether common or different in the young and old.

Culturally appropriate ways of delivering health services

Many services have been developed that broaden the repertoire of provision and help develop partnerships with South Asian communities. One way of working is the specific development of services to provide culturally appropriate services in the desired language. Another is the development of services which, while part of the main service repertoire, are culturally acceptable; for example, dance, gardening and women-only swimming as ways of exercising. Instances of the former include the Bangladeshi Heart Health Project, which is part of the Heartsmart Programme and involves the partnership of two voluntary organisations: the Bangladeshi Porishad and the Bangladeshi Youth Organisation. Another example is the smoking cessation service, which has two South Asian smoking cessation development workers who run a campaign linked with local mosques during Ramadan.

Other examples of culturally appropriate services as part of other services include Asian Men's Health Days, which can be held in local community centres. These deal with issues such as smoking cessation and mental health in a community setting where South Asian men feel more comfortable about discussing health issues. Specific 'Healthwise' courses for Asian women, led by local South Asian workers who are known and respected in the community, have also proved very successful. The women not only successfully complete the course but they support each other and gain the confidence to take part in other health activities. 'Gardening for Health' is a partnership project between the women of the Bangladeshi community, Heartsmart and Bradford Community Environment Project. It won the 1999 National Good Food Award (education category) and it was notable that besides exercise, healthy eating and environmental improvement, the benefits to self-esteem, social interaction and mental health were especially valued.

Increasing the accessibility, acceptability and appropriateness of mainstream services

Strong partnerships between education and health providers have fostered a growing portfolio of activities which bring multiple benefits. Not only has recruitment of South Asian young people to a wide range of health careers increased but the local health services have also gained a more reflective workforce, more confident in demonstrating empathy, curiosity and respect (see, for example, Darr and Bharj, 1999 for a broader discussion of these issues).[3] Further, the health services engaged in this work gain ideas and support to enable them to change their services and introduce more flexible, responsive systems. An excellent example of this includes being flexible when planning services around religious festivals, by using a multi-faith calendar.

Daring to be different

The importance of innovation is evident in many of the effective partnerships to improve health services for South Asian communities. In effect, 'if you do what you've always done, you'll get what you've always got', and this supports the need to do things differently if health outcomes for South Asian populations are to improve. A particularly innovative partnership, which was supported by the Health Action Zone Innovation Programme and several partner health authorities, was the production of 13 half-hour drama, 'soap opera' type programmes set in West Yorkshire entitled 'Kismet Road'. This has involved local people in developing health-related storylines; they also featured as supporting actors in scenes filmed by a professional production company within local health facilities. Although it has attracted some ill-informed newspaper criticism as a poor use of health-related money, the local partnerships have stood firm in their belief in its potential to promote cross-cultural communication as well as its importance for improving health services to South Asian communities. A programme of evaluation will identify how far these expectations will be fulfilled.

Conclusions

Partnerships to improve health services for South Asian communities need to exist at all levels – from one-to-one interactions, through service design and delivery, to strategic planning and interagency working. They need to be evident in research, support of self-help groups, specially targeted and mainstream services. They also need to be based on community development approaches, building long-term relationships and trust between service providers and the communities they serve.

Health service providers need to become representative of the populations they serve and their staff must be supported to practise culturally competent communication, which is informed by empathy, curiosity and respect for all of its users as well as its staff. When this is widely available, each individual will be able to have confidence that their health needs will be identified and met – whatever their ethnic origin – through truly accessible, acceptable and appropriate services.

Modernising services to remove the current problems that hinder cross-cultural communication will initially require more time: more time for one-to-one interaction, more time for staff training and support, more time for sustained work with South Asian communities. In the longer term, however, the gains from better health protection, promotion and improvement are likely to far exceed any costs.

Acknowledgements

Grateful thanks are extended to the many colleagues who supplied so many examples of local work to improve health services for South Asian populations in Bradford. Only a few could be mentioned in the examples section to give a flavour of the approaches used.

References

1 Carrillo JE, Green AR and Betancount JR (1999) Cross-cultural primary care: a patient-based approach. *Annals of Internal Medicine.* **130** (10): 829–34.
2 Department of Health (2002) *The NHS Plan.* HMSO, London.
3 Darr A and Bharj K (1999) Addressing culture diversity in health care: the challenge facing nursing. In: Atkin K, Thompson C and Lunt N (eds) *Evaluating Community Nursing.* Bailliere Tindal, London.

PART 3

Modernising primary care and improving clinical outcomes

CHAPTER 7

Heart disease: an assessment of the importance of socio-economic position

James Nazroo

This chapter is the first exploring specific NHS priorities as defined by National Service Frameworks. Here the focus is one specific health condition: heart disease. The chapter presents empirical material to explore reasons for the higher rate of heart disease among South Asian populations. In doing so it provides a valuable evidence base for those working in primary care. More generally, and bearing in mind Stephen Harrison's concern about the development of services based on specific diseases at the expense of engaging with broader issues of equity, this chapter attempts to locate the experience of South Asian populations within the broader context of ethnicity and health. In doing so, it develops two themes identified in Chapter 2 as relevant to understanding the experience of South Asian people: the importance of not treating South Asian populations as a homogenous group and the value of considering ethnicity within the broader context of socio-economic disadvantage.

These data have led researchers, practitioners and policy makers to ignore socio-economic position when investigating the greater risk of South Asian people for ischaemic heart disease (IHD) and to focus on other possible explanations. Particularly prominent has been the investigation of the role that genetically determined insulin resistance syndrome may play.[1–5] South Asian people have been repeatedly shown to have higher rates of Type 2 diabetes and this is thought to be a consequence of insulin resistance.[2,3] The associated elevated concentration of insulin in plasma is thought to either directly, or through its effects on plasma concentrations of high-density lipoprotein cholesterol and triglycerides, increase the risk of atherosclerosis.[6] Some argue that this biological risk is related to evolutionary processes,[7,8] ethnicity here is used as a marker for biological race. It has also been argued that the increased risk of South Asians for IHD might be related to cultural factors, such as diet and a sedentary lifestyle,[8] although there is little convincing evidence to support these propositions.[6]

More recently, however, an analysis of morbidity rates in the British Fourth National Survey (FNS) suggested variations in risk across South Asian groups. Indian people had rates of heart disease similar to those for the general population, while Pakistani and Bangladeshi people had rates that were more than 80 per cent higher.[9] These morbidity data also showed variations in risk of heart disease across religious groups, with Indian Muslims having higher rates than their Sikh and Hindu counterparts.[9] The implication of these findings is that the aetiological mechanisms leading to a higher risk of IHD for South Asian people are not consistent across the ethnic groups that are included under this label. Indeed, a retrospective examination of some of the earlier immigrant mortality statistics shows that they also suggest a higher risk for those of Muslim origin.[10]

In addition, analysis of British immigrant mortality statistics over the period 1991–93 for men aged 45–64 showed that occupational class is strongly related to risk of death from IHD for men born both on the Indian subcontinent and in East Africa, with those in lower classes at greater risk.[11] A similar pattern was present in the morbidity data collected in the British FNS,[9] but for both the immigrant mortality data and the FNS, standardising for occupational class did not reduce the risk for South Asian people.[9,10] This suggests that although socio-economic position was related to risk of IHD within South Asian groups, as it is for other ethnic groups, it did not contribute to the overall greater risk for South Asian people. However, detailed analysis of the FNS data cast doubt on the usefulness of occupational class as an indicator for socio-economic position when making comparisons across groups. For example, within particular class bands, ethnic minorities were shown to have much lower incomes than white people.[9]

Within this broad context, this chapter presents secondary analysis of morbidity data derived from the British FNS. It builds on work already reported,[9] using multivariate analysis to explore further the higher rates of IHD among South Asian people and the contribution of socio-economic factors to these.

Research methods

The FNS was a representative study of ethnic minority and white people living in England and Wales, conducted in 1993–94. The aim was to describe and explain the experiences of ethnic minority people living in England and Wales. Below is a brief description of the methods used, full details have been published elsewhere.[9,12–14]

The ethnic groups covered are shown in Table 7.1, which also shows numbers and response rates. The allocation of individuals into ethnic groups in the box and the rest of the analysis presented here was based on their response to a question asking about family origins, which very closely correlated with responses to a question on self-assigned ethnic group worded similarly to that used in the 1991

Table 7.1   Composition of respondents to the FNS

Ethnic group	Number of respondents	Response rate (%)
White	2867	71
Caribbean	1205	61
Indian	2001	74
Pakistani	1185	73
Bangladeshi	591	83
Chinese	214	66

Census.[9] The analysis presented here is restricted to the white and South Asian groups. Initial analysis of these data showed that rates of heart disease were similar for Pakistani and Bangladeshi people,[9] so these groups have been combined here. The analysis is also restricted to those aged 40 or older because some of the survey questions on heart disease (which are described later) were asked only of this age group.

Sampling procedures were designed to select probability samples of both individuals and households. Sampling points were identified using information from the 1991 British Census. Areas with both high and low concentrations of ethnic minority people were included to ensure that the sample was, with appropriate weighting, fully representative. Screening for ethnic minority respondents was carried out in the field using a method known as focused enumeration, which has been shown to provide good coverage of the targeted populations.[15,16] This process relies on the visibility of ethnic minority groups, with recruiters identifying households containing ethnic minority people by visiting, for example, every sixth address in a defined area and asking about the ethnic origin of those living at both the visited address and the five addresses on each side (so each non-visited address was asked about twice). Then, if a positive or uncertain identification is made at a visited address for a non-visited address, the recruiter goes on to visit the non-visited address in person. White respondents were identified using a straightforward stratified sampling process, whereby areas, then addresses and then individuals within addresses were identified to be included in the study.

Data were collected using a structured questionnaire. The interview schedule was translated into a variety of South Asian languages and the interview itself was carried out in the language(s) of the respondents' choice. The questions used to identify those with possible heart disease are shown in Box 7.1 and covered both the reporting of a diagnosis of angina or heart disease and the experience of chest pain. The following analysis does not include those reporting chest pain unless it was reported to be 'severe' and had lasted for more than half an hour.[17,18]

The other two key variables used here assessed socio-economic position. Occupational class is based on the employment status and occupation of the head of household, classified according to the British Registrar General's criteria. Standard of living is a composite of housing quality and ownership of consumer durables and was specifically tailored to be sensitive to ethnic differences in socio-economic position.[9] Its composition is shown in Box 7.2.

Box 7.1   Survey questions on heart disease

1   Do you now have or have you ever had angina?
2   Do you now have or have you ever had a heart attack – including a heart murmur, a damaged heart or a rapid heart?
3   [If aged 40 or over and no to both question 1 and 2] Have you ever had any pain or discomfort in your chest?
4   [If 'yes' to question 3] Have you ever had a severe pain across the front of your chest lasting for more than half an hour?

Box 7.2   Standard of living index

This takes into account overcrowded housing, quality of housing and possession of consumer durables and cars.

Poor
- More than one person per room **or**
- Household does not have sole access to one of: a bath or shower; a bathroom; an inside toilet; a kitchen; hot water from a tap; central heating **or**
- Household has less than four consumer durables out of: telephone; video; fridge; freezer; washing machine; tumble-drier; dishwasher; microwave; CD-player; personal computer.

Average
- Those between the good and poor groups.

Good
- Less than 0.75 people per room **and**
- Household has sole access to all housing amenities **and**
- Household has nine or more consumer durables, or five or more consumer durables and access to two or more cars.

On the whole this chapter is concerned with a comparative analysis, but there are limitations with this, as such an approach hides actual rates of illness in communities and absolute greater risks between groups.[9] Consequently, in addition to presenting age-standardised relative risks and odds ratios, where relevant actual rates and absolute greater risks are presented. The age-standardised relative risks and the odds ratios that are reported here are made in comparison with the white group.

Research findings

The absolute per cent columns in Table 7.2 show that men reported higher rates of heart disease than women for each ethnic group and for each stage of questioning. The age-standardised relative risks also showed a consistent pattern across each stage of questioning and for men and women, but not across the two South Asian groups. Pakistani and Bangladeshi people had a higher relative risk compared with white people and this was statistically significant for all but one question (reported heart attack). For Indian people there was little difference compared with white people for each stage of questioning and none of the differences were statistically significant.

Figure 7.1 shows that for each ethnic group the rate of reporting diagnosed heart disease or severe chest pain increased with age. Across the age groups the rate for Pakistani and Bangladeshi respondents remained consistently high, while that for white and Indian people remained very similar. The bars in the figure show relative risks and 95 per cent confidence intervals for the Pakistani and Bangladeshi

Table 7.2 Reported indicators of heart disease and ethnicity B population-based absolute rates and age-standardised relative risk compared with white people (aged 40 or older)

	Pakistani and Bangladeshi		Indian		White
	Absolute per cent	Age-standardised relative risk compared with white people	Absolute per cent	Age-standardised relative risk compared with white people	Absolute per cent
Angina					
Men	11.9	1.92 (1.29–2.86)	6.3	1.13 (0.73–1.75)	8.4
Women	8.6	2.55 (1.56–4.15)	4.2	1.02 (0.58–1.82)	6.4
Heart attack*					
Men	10.9	1.40 (0.96–2.05)	6.8	0.93 (0.62–1.40)	10.2
Women	4.8	1.29 (0.65–2.55)	3.0	0.85 (0.43–1.68)	5.4
Angina or heart attack					
Men	16.6	1.56 (1.13–2.14)	9.4	0.96 (0.67–1.36)	13.9
Women	11.1	1.86 (1.23–2.82)	6.1	0.91 (0.58–1.45)	10.0
Angina, heart attack or severe chest pain					
Men	24.6	1.56 (1.21–2.00)	12.5	0.83 (0.62–1.12)	19.0
Women	22.7	2.31 (1.74–3.08)	12.0	1.11 (0.80–1.54)	14.2

*In addition to 'Heart attack', the question wording added 'including a heart murmur, a damaged heart or a rapid heart'.

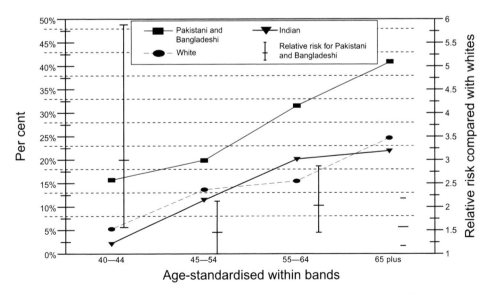

Figure 7.1 Reported heart attack, angina, or severe chest pain: age and ethnicity effects for white and South Asian people.

group and suggest that the younger Pakistani and Bangladeshi respondents had the greatest relative risk. However, absolute risk was greatest for the oldest age group, where the difference between the white and Pakistani and Bangladeshi groups was more than 15 per cent.

Logistic regression analyses were performed to assess the importance of socio-economic factors, with reporting diagnosed heart disease or severe chest pain as the outcome variable. Initially the three ethnic groups were analysed separately to assess whether socio-economic gradients were present within each group. Basic demographic variables (gender, age and age squared) with either occupational class or standard of living were entered into each equation. Both indicators of socio-economic position uncovered a gradient in risk of reported heart disease for each ethnic group similar to findings published elsewhere,[9] with those that were worse off having higher rates.

Following this, two logistic regression analyses were carried out to assess the contribution of socio-economic factors to ethnic differences. The first, shown in Figure 7.2, compared all South Asian respondents with white respondents, so that the findings presented here could be compared with previous analyses of class effects within immigrant mortality statistics. The second, shown in Figure 7.3, compared just Pakistani and Bangladeshi people with white people, as it was this group that Table 7.2 had suggested were at greatest risk. Both figures show odds ratios with 95 per cent confidence intervals, with the first bar showing the odds ratio compared with white people to have reported diagnosed heart disease or severe chest pain without taking into account socio-economic factors, while the following bars show the effect of controlling for occupational class, or standard of living, or both.

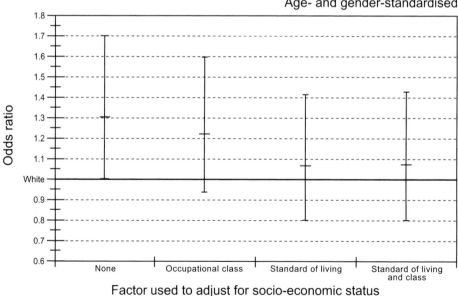

Figure 7.2   Effect of adjusting for socio-economic status on odds ratio of reporting diagnosed heart disease or severe chest pain: South Asian people compared with white people, aged 40–64.

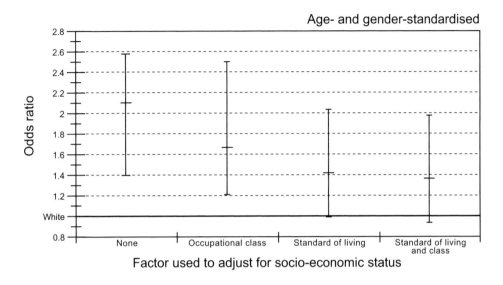

Figure 7.3 Effect of adjusting for socio-economic status on odds ratio of reporting diagnosed heart disease or severe chest pain: Pakistani and Bangladeshi people compared with white people, aged 40–64.

Comparing the first and second bars in the figures shows that controlling for occupational class had only a marginal effect in both cases, although its effect was greater when the Pakistani and Bangladeshi group were considered on their own. However, comparing the third bar with the first in the figures shows that controlling for standard of living leads to a big reduction in the odds ratio, which for all South Asian respondents (Figure 7.2) almost drops to 1, and for Pakistani and Bangladeshi respondents alone (Figure 7.3) drops to a level that is not statistically significant. The final bar in both figures confirms that occupational class adds little to the analysis.

Discussion

The recent analysis of British immigrant mortality statistics has suggested that risk of death from IHD is related to occupational class.[11] The analysis of self-reported morbidity presented here confirms these conclusions. Pakistani and Bangladeshi people, who are on average very poor,[9] had very high rates of reported indicators of heart disease, while Indian people, who have a socio-economic profile closer to that of the general population,[9] had average rates. For each ethnic group studied here (white, Indian, and Pakistani and Bangladeshi), the risk of reported indicators of heart disease was related to socio-economic position, with the better off having lower rates. However, as for the analysis of immigrant mortality rates in Britian,[11] controlling for occupational class made little difference to the greater risk for Pakistani and Bangladeshi people. In the introduction to this chapter, it was suggested that occupational class was an inadequate indicator of socio-economic position when making comparisons across ethnic groups. In the analysis controlling for a more sensitive indicator of ethnic differences in socio-economic position, standard of living greatly reduced the higher risk of reported heart disease found among Pakistani and Bangladeshi respondents. This suggests that, in fact, socio-economic position made an important contribution to the higher rates of heart disease among this group.

Two immediate messages emerge from this analysis. First, socio-economic position should not be ignored when investigating ethnic differences in heart disease: it may make an important contribution to the inequalities that have been reported. Indeed, findings from the FNS have shown that differences in socio-economic position contribute to ethnic inequalities in health across a variety of dimensions.[9] Second, careful thought needs to be given to the adequacy of the indicator of socio-economic position that is used. The common strategy of presenting data that are standardised for an indicator of socio-economic position and then interpreting the resultant difference between ethnic groups as an (unmeasured) ethnic or 'race' effect is not satisfactory. There are a number of statistical and conceptual flaws with such an approach, not least that such measures are rarely equivalent for different ethnic groups, that have been discussed in full in both the British and American literature.[19–21]

There do remain two puzzling inconsistencies, one between the earlier analysis of British immigrant mortality data and that conducted more recently, the other between the more recent British immigrant mortality analysis and the morbidity data presented here. The first concerns the failure to identify a class gradient in the analysis of British data conducted around the 1971 Census.[22] This may be because the downward social mobility of migrant groups when they arrived in Britain in the 1950s and 1960s was not yet fully reflected in the occupations recorded on death certificates in the early 1970s, i.e. some deaths were coded in a higher occupational class than that occupied post-migration to Britain. This inflation of occupational class on death certificates has been noted elsewhere,[23] and, because of the small number of deaths, need only have happened a few times for the figures to have been distorted.

The other concerns the relatively higher mortality rates from IHD among almost all of the South Asian groups in the analysis around the 1991 British Census,[11] compared with the average morbidity rates shown here for Indian people. There are a number of possible explanations for this difference. It might be related to measurement problems both in this and other studies. For example, in mortality data IHD may be over-recorded as a cause of death for those born in South Asia, or in this survey Indian respondents may have under-reported heart disease morbidity. Indeed, there are clearly potential problems with the questions used in the FNS, which rely on self-reports of diagnosis and the experience of chest pain. However, some confidence in the data can be drawn from a number of sources. First, the findings do show a remarkable consistency in response across the different types of questions used to identify heart disease. So, as Table 7.2 shows, questions on diagnosed angina, diagnosed heart attack, chest pain and severe chest pain lasting for more than half an hour showed a very similar pattern across ethnic groups and between men and women within ethnic groups. If there were significant reporting biases, they would not be expected to be consistent across different types of questions.[9] Second, while there is only limited evidence on possible ethnic differences in reporting symptoms, what there is is reassuring. One study, using a vignette, has suggested that South Asian and white people interpret chest pain similarly.[24]

Of course, morbidity and mortality rates need not necessarily entirely co-vary. In this case, the morbidity rates covered prevalence, while the mortality rates covered incidence and survival, and rates of survival might vary across different ethnic groups because of differences in the quality of treatment received. It has been shown that among those suffering a myocardial infarction rates of admission to hospital are related to area deprivation scores,[25] and, among those who have suffered an acute myocardial infarction one study has suggested that Indian patients are less likely to be treated with thrombolysis[26] or to be referred for exercise stress tests.[27] Similar findings have been reported in the United States.[28–30] In addition, ethnic differences in the progression of the disease might be important. In another study, although white and South Asian patients admitted to hospital with a myocardial infarction received very similar treatment, the South Asian patients had a higher case fatality rate than the white patients, perhaps because of a higher co-morbidity with diabetes.[31]

All of this highlights the importance of considering multifactorial explanations for the higher rate of IHD in some South Asian groups. Explanations that emphasise only one risk factor may fail to identify the inter-relationships between different risk factors. Particularly important is that an exclusive focus on genetic or biological explanations ignores: the importance of environmental triggers for genetic risk; that biological markers may be the consequence of environmental exposure rather than genetic risk; and that ethnicity or 'race' may be a marker for social disadvantage leading to increased risk. This, then, may lead to important points of intervention being missed.

Acknowledgements

This chapter is an abridged version of a paper initially published in *Ethnicity and Disease*, **11** (3): 401–11. The study on which the chapter is based was undertaken jointly by the Policy Studies Institute and Social and Community Planning Research. I am grateful to my colleagues from both institutions who worked with me on the FNS, particularly Sharon Beishon, Richard Berthoud, Tariq Modood, Gillian Prior, Patten Smith and Satnam Virdee. I am also grateful to David Halpern, who developed the health elements of the FNS questionnaire. The work on which this chapter is based was supported by a grant from the (UK) Economic and Social Research Council under the Health Variations Programme (L128251019).

References

1   Knight TM, Smith Z, Whittles A *et al.* (1992) Insulin resistance, diabetes, and risk markers for ischaemic heart disease in Asian men and non-Asian men in Bradford. *British Heart Journal.* **67**: 343–50.

2   McKeigue P, Marmot M, Syndercombe Court Y *et al.* (1988) Diabetes, hyperinsulinaemia, and coronary risk factors in Bangladeshis in East London. *British Heart Journal.* **60**: 390–6.

3   McKeigue P, Shah B and Marmot M (1991) Relation of central obesity and insulin resistance with high diabetes prevalence and cardiovascular risk in South Asians. *Lancet.* **337**: 382–6.

4   McKeigue P (1992) Coronary heart disease in Indians, Pakistanis and Bangladeshis: aetiology and possibilities for prevention. *British Heart Journal.* **67**: 341–2.

5   Shaukat N and Cruickshank J (1993) Coronary artery disease: impact upon black and ethnic minority people. In: Hopkins A and Bahl V (eds) *Access to Health Care for People from Black and Ethnic Minorities*, pp. 133–46. Royal College of Physicians, London.

6   McKeigue P, Miller G and Marmot M (1989) Coronary heart disease in South Asians overseas: a review. *Journal of Clinical Epidemiology*. **42** (7): 597–609.

7   McKeigue P and Sevak L (1994) *Coronary Heart Disease in South Asian Communities*. Health Education Authority, London.

8   Gupta S, de Belder A and O'Hughes L (1995) Avoiding premature coronary deaths in Asians in Britain: spend now on prevention or pay later for treatment. *BMJ*. **311**: 1035–6.

9   Nazroo JY (1997) *The Health of Britain's Ethnic Minorities: findings from a national survey*. Policy Studies Institute, London.

10   Balarajan R, Bulusu L, Adelstein AM *et al.* (1984) Patterns of mortality among migrants to England and Wales from the Indian subcontinent. *BMJ*. **289**: 1185–7.

11   Harding S and Maxwell R (1997) Differences in the mortality of migrants. In: Drever F and Whitehead M (eds) *Health Inequalities*. Decennial supplement series DS no. 15. The Stationery Office, London.

12   Smith P and Prior G (1996) *The Fourth National Survey of Ethnic Minorities: technical report*. Social and Community Planning Research, London.

13   Modood T, Berthoud R, Lakey J *et al.* (1997) *Ethnic Minorities in Britain: diversity and disadvantage*. Policy Studies Institute, London.

14   Nazroo JY (1997) *Ethnicity and Mental Health: findings from a national community survey*. Policy Studies Institute, London.

15   Brown C and Ritchie J (1981) *Focused Enumeration: the development of a method for sampling ethnic minority groups*. Policy Studies Institute/SCPR, London.

16   Smith P (1996) Methodological aspects of research amongst ethnic minorities. *Survey Methods Centre Newsletter*. **16** (1): 20–4.

17   Rose GA and Blackburn H (1986) *Cardiovascular Survey Methods*. World Health Organization, Geneva.

18   Erens B and Primatesta P (1999) *Health Survey for England: cardiovascular disease*. The Stationery Office, London.

19   Bhopal R (1997) Is research into ethnicity and health racist, unsound, or important science? *BMJ*. **314**: 1751–6.

20   Kauffman JS, Cooper RS and McGee DL (1997) Socio-economic status and health in blacks and whites: the problem of residual confounding and the resiliency of race. *Epidemiology*. **8** (6): 621–8.

21   Morgenstern H (1997) Defining and explaining race effects. *Epidemiology*. **8** (6): 609–11

22   Marmot MG, Adelstein AM, Bulusu L *et al.* (1984) *Immigrant Mortality in England and Wales 1970–78: causes of death by country of birth*. HMSO, London.

23   Townsend P and Davidson N (1982) *Inequalities in Health (the Black Report)*. Penguin, Harmondsworth.

24   Chaturvedi N, Rai H and Ben-Shlomo Y (1997) Lay diagnosis and health care-seeking behaviour for chest pain in South Asians and Europeans. *Lancet*. **350**: 1578–83.

25   Mackenback JP, Looman CW and van der Meer JB (1996) Differences in the misreporting of chronic conditions by level of education: the effect on inequalities in prevalence rates. *American Journal of Public Health.* **86** (5): 706–11.

26   Blane D, Power C and Bartley M (1996) Illness behaviour and the measurement of class differentials in morbidity. *Journal of the Royal Statistical Society.* **156** (Part 1): 77–92.

27   Morrison C, Woodward M, Leslie W *et al.* (1997) Effect of socio-economic group on incidence of, management of, and survival after myocardial infarction and coronary death: analysis of community coronary event register. *BMJ.* **314**: 541–6.

28.   Lear JT, Lawrence IG, Pohl JE *et al.* (1994) Myocardial infarction and thrombolysis: a comparison of the Indian and European populations on a coronary care unit. *Journal of the Royal College of Physicians.* **28** (2): 143–7.

29   Lear JT, Lawrence IG, Burden AC *et al.* (1994) A comparison of stress test referral rates and outcome between Asians and Europeans. *Journal of the Royal Society of Medicine.* **87** (11): 661–2.

30   Wenneker MB and Epstein AM (1989) Racial inequalities in the use of procedures for patients with ischaemic heart disease in Massachusetts. *Journal of the American Medical Association.* **261** (2): 253–7.

31   Whittle J, Conigliaro J, Good CB *et al.* (1993) Racial differences in the use of invasive cardiovascular procedures in the Department of Veterans Affairs medical system. *New England Journal of Medicine.* **329** (9): 621–7.

CHAPTER 8

Mental health: disadvantage, discrimination and distress

Sashi Sashidharan and Martin Commander

Mental health has long been a feature of the broader debates about ethnicity and health. It is an area where there has been considerable activity, although this has not always been for the benefit of minority ethnic populations. This chapter outlines the extent of mental health problems amongst people of South Asian origin living in the UK, possible determinants of their psychiatric morbidity and an overview of how the mental healthcare needs of this community are being addressed within current provisions of the NHS. In doing so, the chapter applies many of the ideas presented in Chapter 2 and identifies a number of key theoretical and empirical issues which, it is argued, are relevant when considering the mental health needs of people of South Asian origin living in the UK, especially within primary care.

Defining ethnicity

Ethnicity, as we have seen in Chapter 2, is a problematic concept, both as a way of establishing or attributing identity or when categorising populations. This seems particularly to be the case when considering the health of minority groups, defined according to their 'ethnicity'.[1] By exploring some of the themes identified in Chapter 2, this chapter will begin by critically evaluating current understanding and argue this must be the starting point in any debate about improving mental health outcomes for South Asian populations. Often, for example, the extent of the imprecision inherent in ethnic categorisation and the lack of empirical or theoretical underpinnings for such categorisation are rarely acknowledged within research or when developing health policies and services. In addition, few health benefits appear to follow from the focus on ethnicity within the healthcare field. There is a long history of research and discourse around ethnicity and health in this country. There is, however, little evidence that the healthcare of minority ethnic groups in this country has improved as a result of such professional and academic interest. Furthermore, it could be argued that ethnic health research itself may be part of a process of pathologising ethnic minorities rather than addressing apparent inequities in health and health service experience. The fundamental problem here is that research in relation to ethnicity or 'race' has been predominantly concerned with ethnic variations in disease rates and disease manifestations to the relative exclusion of the social and material factors that have a bearing on health and healthcare. This preoccupation with ethnic differences in disease manifestation is further evidence of the academic and theoretical bias towards sustaining a quasi-scientific basis for racial typologies and the notion of 'race' difference.[2]

Notwithstanding these conceptual and ethical problems, it could be argued that 'ethnicity', in a given political and cultural context, signifies the differential positions, experiences and, to a lesser extent, identities within a multicultural population (see also Chapter 2). When applied to the differential experience of the population, say in relation to the use of health services, it can tell us something about the way inequalities exist within service provisions and the institutional bias that underpins such inequity. In other words, ethnicity, like gender or income or class, can be a useful tool in explaining the discrepancies and the unequal access and outcome that exist within the health service. As many other chapters in this book demonstrate, ethnicity is not always the key variable. However, there is a further problem when ethnic categories are understood as an inclusive and general description relating to historically determined but nonetheless commonsensical differentiation of a culturally diverse population. Within the collective experience of such broadly defined demographic categories, significant and often useful differences are not usually made visible. This is most telling when we consider ethnic groups as they are defined and understood in contemporary discourses in Britain. In order to understand the extent and nature of such differences we are required to drill down further within the broader ethnic categories and seek more specific associations and cultural experiences within less diverse populations such as South Asian, Indian, Pakistani, African Caribbean, Black, Chinese and Irish. Although the political nature of who gets officially defined as 'ethnic' in England is recognised, the categories here follow the major ethnicity categories used in the Census 2001, which in turn form common standards for research and monitoring. The Census 2001 (www.census.org.uk) differentiated Irish people in England for the first time from the 'white' category. It is accepted that many other 'white' ethnic groups, including Poles, Italians, Greek Cypriots and Turkish Cypriots, continue to be made invisible at official level.

Mental health policy

There are good reasons for being concerned with the mental health problems of different minority ethnic groups in England. First and foremost, ethnicity is a critical factor that needs to be taken into account when planning and delivering mental health services in a multicultural community. This might seem self-evident but the history of mental health policy and service development in England tells a different story. Until recently, policy development in mental health at the national level and service developments locally have rarely paid adequate attention to the specific and variable needs of the various minority ethnic groups living in this country. This should now be a familiar theme.

Although the extent and nature of the difficulties and disadvantages experienced by black and minority ethnic groups within mental health services have been recognised for a long time, the evidence to date is that these ethnic differences in service experience and outcome are persisting and, if anything, are getting worse. Results from two recent surveys, for example, confirm that black and minority ethnic groups continue to experience major problems in accessing mental health services that are appropriate to their needs. The overall care experience is reported as uniformly negative.[3,4] There are, however, no nationally co-ordinated plans or actions intended specifically to address these problems. Both professionally and politically there appears to be a singular lack of commitment to engage with black and minority ethnic groups in addressing their mental health problems or in dealing with the ethnic bias in service provisions. Clearly, there is a need for a coherent national strategy to make mental health services more sensitive and appropriate to the needs of multicultural Britain.

In spite of this, there are grounds for optimism. Mental health services in England are currently undergoing a period of significant change. For the first time, mental health is now identified as a clinical priority within the NHS. The National Service Framework and the National Plan for Mental Health provide a set of priorities and an action plan for the development of progressive mental health services, underpinned by clear values and a commitment to improve the quality of services in general. These innovations in policy and service development have also created a readiness to reappraise the nature of mental health problems and the scope and limitations of conventional treatment options. For example, a broader psychosocial approach is becoming more visible within the current attempts to improve services. There is also an explicit acknowledgement that social and material conditions could have an impact on the emergence of mental ill health as well as influencing service interventions and their outcome. As a result, ethnicity, along with social marginalisation and social exclusion, are likely to assume a greater importance within the reform agenda for mental health services than has been the case so far.[5]

Political context and institutional racism

Allied to these developments within mental health policy and service developments in the recent years, ethnicity and the broader concerns around social exclusion are beginning to find clearer articulation within both governmental and professional circles. For example, specific actions are being planned to combat discrimination and inequality within the health service. Following the Stephen Lawrence inquiry, it is now acknowledged that the NHS, like other public bodies in this country, is institutionally racist (see Chapter 2). As we have seen, recommendations arising out of the Lawrence inquiry have had a far-reaching effect on public services in general and government as well as professional thinking. As a result there is now a greater willingness in addressing the needs of minority ethnic groups and to reappraise the nature of their experiences within public services such as the NHS. Whether this will result in a political commitment to challenge the ethnic inequities that exist within the health service, in particular mental health services, however, remains unclear.

One of the key recommendations arising out of the Lawrence inquiry is that it is important to address the problems experienced by black and minority ethnic groups within our public services through changes in the organisational culture, institutional reforms and policies rather than through marginal attempts to improve the ethnic sensitivity of services or service providers. By placing institutional racism at the heart of the debate around the relationship between minority ethnic groups and public services in this country, as well as within the general discourse on race relations, the Macpherson report (1999)[6] has made a significant advance in our thinking. This has made it possible to reform the institutional agencies with clear objectives and programmes around equality of opportunity and outcome.

The introduction of the Race Relations (Amendment) Act (2000), as Chapter 2 argues, is particularly significant in this context. As the Act sets out, it is no longer necessary to prove intent to establish racial discrimination. Public bodies are, as a result, charged with the responsibility to ensure that their interventions or services do not result in disparities in outcome. The responsibility to monitor outcomes according to ethnicity and take appropriate steps to eradicate racial discrimination rests with the organisations concerned. All public bodies, including those providing and commissioning healthcare, are bound by these requirements.[7]

The changing discourse around ethnicity and mental health

The relationship between ethnicity and mental health has been the focus of much debate and dispute in this country for several years now. Over the recent past this debate has moved on, from earlier preoccupations with *race differences* and ethnic or cultural *predispositions* to mental illness, to considering the *aversive experiences* of black and minority ethnic groups in contemporary British society and its institutions, including mental health services. There have been three significant changes in the debates and discourse around 'race' or ethnicity within mental health services.

- First, the earlier preoccupation around ethnic vulnerability to mental diseases, as shown in research studies concerned with establishing differential rates of, mostly, severe mental illness according to ethnicity, appears to be diminishing. One of the reasons for this is the recognition that such research is often flawed, both methodologically and conceptually, and the research findings have added little of value to our understanding of mental disorders in general or the mental health experience of minority ethnic groups in particular.
- Secondly, there is now a greater willingness to consider the psychosocial determinants and the material context of mental health difficulties among minority ethnic groups. In other words, the priority previously attributed to race, culture or ethnicity in accounting for ethnic variations in disease manifestation, clinical practice, health service experience and outcome is, to some extent, challenged by linking such differences more clearly to material and social conditions, in particular the social exclusion and material inequalities.
- Thirdly, there has been a welcome shift both within research and in clinical services from a preoccupation with ethnic differences in disease manifestation and the presumed cultural or ethnic roots of illness to how the mental health problems of minority ethnic groups ought to be managed in an appropriate and acceptable manner. This is particularly important when addressing the long-established ethnic inequalities in the service experience and the ethnically discrepant outcomes of healthcare interventions. In this context, the totality of the mental health experience of minority groups is the subject of study rather than particular disease conditions that are often allied to specific ethnic or cultural groups.

The experience of the mental health of ethnic minorities, therefore, is increasingly acknowledged as being closely linked to their wider experiences of disadvantage and discrimination in the UK. According to such an analysis, the marginality and social exclusion of minority ethnic groups are critical in providing meaningful understanding of the mental health of people in these communities and their differential access to mental health services and experiences within it. This experience of discrimination and disadvantage is characterised by diversity between and within ethnic groups, and this complexity needs to be borne in mind when addressing the needs of black and minority ethnic groups in general. Like the majority white population, gender, social class, age, geography and migration status mediate the healthcare experience of minority groups (see also Chapter 2). To a large extent, wider structural inequalities account for the mental health experience of Britain's minorities. Such disadvantages, which disproportionately affect minorities, are partly caused by racism and discrimination in all areas of social life, including the mental health system. Any strategy that aims to address ethnic inequalities in the healthcare experience and health outcomes needs be based on an understanding of the specific requirements and backgrounds of the ethnic groups as well as the culture of the health service itself.

For these reasons, we will now deal with the social and material circumstances of minority ethnic groups with particular reference to South Asian people before considering the nature of mental health problems in this community and some of the difficulties identified in their service experience. For this purpose, we rely on the findings of a series of surveys that were carried out in an inner-city district in Birmingham, with a culturally diverse population. We present our findings based on studies carried out at the individual level but relating the actual experience of the health service by minority ethnic groups to the broader findings emerging on the basis of national surveys concerning the social and material conditions of South Asian people. It is important to link the findings from individual surveys with the broader picture of the socio-demographic position of South Asian populations in this country if we are to seek appropriate and effective strategies to reduce the burden of mental ill health in this community and bring about meaningful changes in the way services are currently organised and delivered. To this extent, we identify important contextual features, which should inform any analysis of a given health problem among South Asian populations.

Making sense of mental health among South Asian populations

A profile of South Asian populations in the UK

According to the latest census, the size of the minority ethnic population in the UK is estimated to be 4.6 million. This constitutes 7.9 per cent of the total population. This proportion would be higher if white Irish people were included amongst minority ethnic groups. South Asian populations are the largest minority ethnic group, with people of Indian, Pakistani and Bangladeshi origin constituting 3.6 per cent of the total population or half of the total minority ethnic population. It is estimated that there are over two million people who are designated as Asian or British Asian living in this country.

Black and ethnic minority populations tend to have a younger age profile than that of the white majority. This is, partly, a reflection of migration and historical patterns of settlement in this country. Nearly half (48 per cent) of the minority ethnic population is under 24 years old, compared with 31 per cent of the white population. Bangladeshis in particular have a comparatively young population. Thirty eight per cent are under 16 years old, double the proportion of the white group. Overall, South Asian households tend to be larger than average, with Bangladeshi households being the largest. Such households may contain three generations living with a married couple and their children. The different demographic structures, cultural traditions and economic characteristics of the South Asian communities underlie distinctive patterns of family size and household compositions. South Asian people are also least likely to live in lone parent families, only nine per cent of Indian and 15 per cent of Pakistani families are lone parent compared to 23 per cent for the white population.

The latest census also reveals the extent of the socio-economic disadvantage experienced by minority ethnic groups in general and South Asian people in particular (see also Chapter 2). There are significant and enduring social and material inequalities between the black and minority ethnic population and the majority white population in Britain. People identifying themselves as of Pakistani and Bangladeshi origin belong to some of the most socially disadvantaged communities in this country. Minority ethnic groups are more likely than the rest of the population to be poor. Measuring household income is the fairest means to assess access to resources as it adjusts for family size. People from minority ethnic groups are more likely to live in low-income households with over 60 per cent of the one million people of Pakistani and Bangladeshi communities living in such households, compared to only 16 per cent of the white community. Bangladeshis have the lowest economic activity rates among both men (69 per cent) and women (22 per cent) compared to 85 per cent for white men and 74 per cent for white women. People of Indian and Pakistani origin are also more likely to be economically inactive when compared to white people. For both men and women from all minority ethnic groups, rates of unemployment are much higher than for white people, with Bangladeshi men showing the highest unemployment rate (20 per cent) – four times that for white men. The unemployment rate is much higher among young people aged less than 25 years in all minority ethnic groups. Pakistani and Bangladeshi men who are unemployed are also likely to have partners who are out of work. People from these two communities, when they are in employment, are more likely to be doing manual jobs compared to white people and those of Indian origin. Educationally Pakistani and Bangladeshi communities appear to be more disadvantaged than all other ethnic groups, a lower proportion of people having educational qualifications and fewer boys and girls from these backgrounds achieving five or more GCSEs (22 and 37 per cent respectively) compared to all other ethnic groups.

Black and minority ethnic groups are more likely than majority white people to live in areas of high social deprivation and poor social cohesion. Minority ethnic people are disproportionately represented in deprived areas and urban areas. Over two-thirds live in London and the three large metropolitan areas in the West Midlands, Greater Manchester and West Yorkshire. In contrast, these areas account for less than a quarter of the white population.

There is a well-established link between structural inequality and variations in health status in all communities. Generally, people from minority ethnic groups in England experience much worse health than the white majority. The findings of the Fourth National Survey of Ethnic Minorities confirm this. Minority ethnic groups, relative to the white majority in England, are more likely to report fair, poor or very poor health, limiting long-standing illness and registered disability as well as significantly higher scores of psychological distress, poor self-assessed general health and severe lack of social support.[8] The survey findings confirm persistent ethnic differences in health status. For example, the prevalence of limiting long-standing illness is higher for Pakistani, Bangladeshi and Irish men and Black Caribbean and South Asian women than for the general population, with risk of poor health increasing among individuals from poorest households. All South Asian groups showed higher rates of most cardiovascular conditions than the general population with Bangladeshis and Pakistanis having higher rates than Indians.

The link between variations in health status and structural inequality has been replicated in studies examining the relationship between unemployment, poverty and social class and rates of common mental disorders.[9] It has been argued that as a consequence of the very high levels of socio-economic deprivation in minority ethnic communities they will show higher rates of mental illness.[10] Indeed, this was confirmed in the community-based surveys that we carried out in Birmingham.[11] Somewhat surprisingly, however, the latest national survey of ethnic minority psychiatric illness rates in the community (EMPIRIC) found only relatively modest differences in morbidity rates across ethnic groups in England.[12] The authors postulate that variables such as housing, employment and education may fail to tap into the key aspects of disadvantage experienced by ethnic minorities. Alternatively, they tentatively propose that the impact of social and material stresses could be moderated by other unadjusted factors such as social support or community social capital. However, the EMPIRIC study failed to find a clear relationship between support and morbidity[13] and indeed highlighted in the qualitative phase of the project a perceived causal role for stressful family relationships. More significantly, they found that experiences of racism were central to the accounts of non-whites with common mental disorders.[14]

Discrimination

The experience of racism and racial discrimination is likely to have a specific bearing on the health status of all ethnic minority groups.[15,16] Racial discrimination is a facet of the lives of all Britain's minorities, and the experience of racial discrimination or racism is likely to be one of the most important determinants of the disadvantaged social and economic positioning of minorities described above. The experience of minority groups within education, in employment, housing and, more generally, in relation to public institutions and services confirms the extent to which institutional racism plays a critical role in perpetuating inequality. Both covert and direct racial discrimination as well as racist attitudes and behaviour have an impact on the health of minority groups (see Chapter 2). In this context, it is not only appropriate but essential to consider racism as an important influence on the health of minority ethnic groups. However, experience of discrimination, by its very nature, is likely to be underestimated in research and epidemiological studies. The difficulties associated with measuring or quantifying the extent of racial discrimination are well known.

Disadvantaged social class position is often taken as evidence of discriminatory racist practice against Black and Asian populations. For example, employment experience is a common nexus around which exclusionary practices operate against many ethnic and migrant groups in Britain. Modood *et al.* (1997)[17] have documented perceived experiences of discrimination in employment against 'visible' minorities. Poorer health may be linked to class position via material and psychosocial pathways and it is important to establish the relationship of discrimination to employment. Black and minority ethnic groups consistently expect to be treated worse by public services than white people and they experience significant levels of harassment within the workplace.

The more prevalent experiences of individual racism and racist incidents are also important in this context. In spite of the problems associated with the reporting of racist incidents there has been a renewed commitment to taking racist incidents seriously, especially by the police, in recent years. The risk of being a victim of a racially motivated incident is considerably higher for members of minority ethnic groups than for white people. The highest risk is for Pakistani and Bangladeshi people at 4.2 per cent, followed by 3.6 per cent for Indian people and 2.2 per cent for black people. This compares with 0.3 per cent for white people. Racially motivated incidents represent 12 per cent of all crimes against minority ethnic people compared with 2 per cent for white people. The British Crime Survey,[18] which provided these figures, also examined the impact of racially motivated incidents on the victims. Emotional reactions to racially motivated incidents were generally more severe than for non-racially motivated incidents. Forty-two per cent of victims of racially motivated crime reported that they were 'very much affected' by the incident compared with 19 per cent of victims of other sorts of crime.

Differential access to mental healthcare

We now explore empirical research on ethnicity and mental health in Birmingham, carried out in the last ten years. The main purpose of this research was to first, provide detailed estimates of psychological disorders at various levels in the pathway to specialist mental healthcare and, second, explore any ethnic differences in the overall population prevalence as well as in the various stages of care pathway, including detection rates in primary care and consequent referrals to specialist care services. This aspect of the study was an attempt to understand the organisational and institutional influences on case detection and referral and the ethnic differences in case rates found at the various stages within the care pathway (*see* Table 8.1).[11,19]

A series of surveys were undertaken in specialist psychiatric settings as well as in primary care and at the general population level. There is a predominance of severe mental illness (schizophrenia and manic depression) within psychiatric settings whereas most morbidity identified in the community consists of affective disorders (depressive and neurotic disorders). The implications for service provision are distinctly different for these two broad diagnostic groupings, which will therefore be considered separately.

The results are comparable to those reported previously[19] and show rates of morbidity diminishing rapidly through successively higher levels of care, with most psychiatric morbidity being managed in general practice (*see* Table 8.1). The differential access to mental healthcare for South Asian populations as compared to white people, consistent with findings from previous UK studies, is clearly

Table 8.1   One-month prevalence rates in the pathways to care

Level	Survey	Method	Morbidity rates*	
			South Asian	White
4 Psychiatric service use**	Specialist services survey	Case register	30	47
Filter 3: decision to refer			*36.9*	*16.4*
3 Primary care: conspicuous morbidity	Primary care survey	GP rating	1108	771
Filter 2: case recognition			*2.7*	*2.0*
2 Primary care: total morbidity	Primary care survey	GHQ-30***	2960	1542
Filter 1: decision to consult			*1.3*	*1.8*
1 Community	General population survey	GHQ-30	3720	2740

* Rates/10 000.
** Restricted to depressive and neurotic disorders.
*** General Health Questionnaire[20] – 30 item version.

demonstrated.[21] South Asian people were more likely to have a mental health problem than other ethnic groups in the general population and were also more likely than others to consult their GPs, but were subsequently less likely to have their problem identified and to be referred on to specialist psychiatric services. Similar results emerged when the analyses were repeated separately for men and women.[22]

In addition to the GHQ-30, the general population survey included a semi-structured mental state interview, the Structured Clinical Interview for DSM IIIR (SCID),[23] to assess affective disorders (major depression, dysthymia, panic disorder, agoraphobia and generalised anxiety disorder) during the previous six months. For those reporting any disorder, help seeking was ascertained.

People, in general, did not report seeking support from alternative healers or priests. They were also less likely than white people to discuss their problem with a relative or friend (*see* Table 8.2). Consistent with the overall findings, they were more likely to consult their GP than white people and were equally likely to discuss their problems. What they disclosed cannot be ascertained from these data but given their willingness to ascribe their problems to psychosocial factors and in many cases attribute them to life events and relationship difficulties it seems likely, as has been noted elsewhere,[24,25] that given the opportunity they would have talked about the emotional nature of their problems. However, half of those who saw their GP (regardless of ethnicity) did not disclose their problems. There is

Table 8.2 Explanation and help seeking

	South Asian n = 33		White n = 44		
	n	Per cent	n	Per cent	
What, if anything, did you think was the matter?					NS
psychosocial problem	22	67	27	61	
physical problem	8	24	5	11	
other or no explanation	3	9	12	27	
What did you think was the likely cause?					NS
psychosocial reason	14	42	22	50	
physical illness	12	36	10	23	
other or no explanation	7	21	12	27	
Discussed problem with a relative/friend	23	70	39	89	$P = 0.04$
Contact with general practitioner	31	94	31	71	$P = 0.01$
Discussed problem with general practitioner*	18	55	16	36	NS

NS = not significant.
* i.e. 58 per cent of Asians and 52 per cent of whites who saw their GP considered that they had discussed their mental health problems.

evidence that people do not see depression as a medical problem, especially where external causal factors are involved.[26] This may be true of the white people in this study, including those who did not consult with their GP but sought support from a confidante. Likewise, South Asian people who see their GP ostensibly for a physical complaint may recognise an emotional component to their problems but simply may not envisage the GP being able to help.[27] It is also possible that many GPs are uneasy about medicalising social difficulties, which they doubt are amenable to medical treatment, especially where other disposal options are lacking.

Further examination of the primary care data reaffirms that South Asian consulters with mental health problems (identified using the GHQ-30) are under-detected by GPs (odds ratios = 0.31, $P = 0.02$) and indeed that they are more likely than white people to be diagnosed incorrectly ($P = 0.02$).[28] Multivariate analyses indicate that these differences are likely to be at least partially explained by differences in clinical presentation rather than due to stereotyping by GPs. The tendency for South Asian people to focus on physical health problems found in this study is in keeping with an extensive research literature documenting that people from the Asian subcontinent 'somatise' their psychological distress.[27] GPs are hindered in their case identification by the presence of physical problems and more effective in identifying those reporting social difficulties or having a history of help-seeking for a psychiatric disorder.[28] Even where GPs do identify morbidity it is clear that filter 3 (referral to psychiatric services) is particularly impermeable to South Asian people. Furthermore, once within specialist mental healthcare settings there continue to be differences in the nature of the service received.

As can be seen from the psychiatric survey data presented in Table 8.3,[29] once within specialist mental health services, Indian and Pakistani patients with both affective disorders and severe mental illness have greater levels of contact with psychiatrists than those from other ethnic groups. As these patients are less likely to be involved with other mental health staff, especially psychologists, it is probable that the service available is predominantly clinic based and prescriptive. This reinforces long-standing unease that black and ethnic minorities are less likely than white people to receive psychosocial interventions.

As mentioned earlier, most morbidity identified in the community consists of affective disorders whereas there is an increasing proportion with severe mental illness within psychiatric settings (*see* Table 8.4). At level 4 (total psychiatric services) 46 per cent have a diagnosis of schizophrenia or manic depression, at level 5 (admission) this rises to 61 per cent and at level 6 (compulsory admission) to 74 per cent. This distinction has a striking impact on the permeability of the third (referral) and fourth (admission) filters. The ratio of level 3 to 4 increased from 6 to 21 and for level 4 to 5 from 13 to 28 when morbidity within psychiatric services was restricted to affective disorders, i.e. filters 3 and 4 were far less permeable to people with these conditions. A comparison of the pathways at this higher level reveals little difference between South Asian and white people, in terms of the permeability of the filters. This is consistent with the limited literature in this area.[21] If anything there is a tendency for South Asian people to be less likely to access inpatient services and to be detained under the Mental Health Act 1983.

In a later study, we specifically examined the ethnic variation in the experience and outcome of specialist mental health interventions surrounding hospital.[30] We looked at the care pathways to the hospital, inpatient and after care for equal numbers of Asian, black and white patients with non-affective psychoses. The most striking finding was the variation in complexity of the pathways to inpatient care. The pathways for most white patients were relatively straightforward whereas only a minority of South Asian patients was admitted after one consultation and many followed tortuous routes, often involving the police. This was despite a similar level of involvement of psychiatric staff and higher levels of contact with their GP. South Asian people were at least as likely as white people to be living with others, discounting the role of social isolation contributing to delay and more aversive entry into inpatient care. Likewise, the psychiatric survey undertaken as part of the earlier research[29] found that Indian and Pakistani patients were more often married and living with others, including children, than other ethnic groups. Furthermore, less than one in ten Indian and Pakistani patients with a severe mental illness were living in communal establishments (hostels and residential homes) compared to a quarter of patients from other ethnic groups. Where differences did emerge were in findings that South Asian patients were significantly less likely than white people to perceive themselves as having a mental health problem and needing to come to a psychiatric hospital. Not surprisingly, they expressed greater dissatisfaction with the process of hospital admission compared with white patients.

Table 8.3   Patterns of psychiatric service use by diagnostic group

	Severe mental illness						Affective disorders					
	Black Caribbean (n = 319)	Indian (n = 100)	Pakistani (n = 34)	Irish (n = 75)	White (n = 462)		Black Caribbean (n = 54)	Indian (n = 61)	Pakistani (n = 41)	Irish (n = 64)	White (n = 418)	
Psychologist	5	4	0	8	4	NS	8	3	2	12	13	P = 0.03
Social worker	21	6	6	16	16	P = 0.009	15	8	13	3	5	P = 0.01
Community psychiatric nurse	25	13	22	25	26	NS	39	17	18	28	35	P = 0.008
Psychiatrist	56	71	66	49	59	P = 0.03	33	62	63	50	40	P = 0.008

Missing data for each variable in any one ethnic group ranged from 0–44 for psychosis/bipolar and from 0–11 for depressive/neurosis and did not exceed 10 per cent.

Table 8.4   Six-month prevalence rates within specialist psychiatric services

Level	Survey	Method	Morbidity rates*	
			South Asian	White
6 Compulsory admission	Specialist services survey	Case register	37	48
Filter 5: use of Mental Health Act			*4.0*	*4.8*
5 Inpatient care	Specialist services survey	Case register	147	228
Filter 4: decision to admit			*9.1*	*8.4*
4 Psychiatric service use	Specialist services survey	Case register	1332	1919

*Rates/100 000.

Discussion

The literature on mental health of South Asian people living in England is con-clusive; like other minority ethnic groups in this country they have much poorer experience of mental health services compared to the majority ethnic group and there are significant and persistent barriers that they encounter at all levels within the care pathway and care systems. This finding is similar to that found in other areas of healthcare where despite high levels of ill health and disability, minority ethnic groups appear to have poorer access to services. For example, South Asian patients are less likely to receive appropriate treatment with lipid-lowering drugs although they have a higher risk of heart disease.[31] They are also less likely to receive appropriate medical care or advice for angina[32] and to undergo invasive management of coronary disease.[33] Much has been made in the literature about the ethnic variations of illness presentation and even in disease rates but, arguably, the most significant observation in this area is that minority ethnic groups in general have a less favourable experience of health services compared to white people. In terms of service improvement and clinical practice this presents us with practical challenges as well as possible remedies in dealing with such inequality.

The prevalence of mental health problems in South Asian communities appears to be higher than for other ethnic groups, including white people. This is not surprising given the very high levels of social, material and economic disadvant-age experienced by South Asian populations in this country. In addition, South Asian people in general experience very high levels of racism, both at the insti-tutional and individual level, which in all likelihood has an adverse impact on their mental health as well as their capacity to deal with health problems. In a recent study of community perspectives on mental health issues in an African Caribbean community, social exclusion was repeatedly invoked as an explanatory framework in understanding the interactions with the mental health services.[34] This is similar to the community perspectives on the experience of mental distress and the negative impact that mental health services have on South Asian people.[35] The high levels of psychological distress found in ethnic minority communities, whilst being linked to the experience of marginality and exclusion, are also mediated through the discrimination and disempowerment that they experience within their interactions with public services and welfare agencies.

At the primary care level there is evidence of systematic under-recognition of psychological distress amongst South Asian people and they follow adverse and complex care pathways before they receive specialist attention.[21] This ethnic inequality in service experience is likely to be a product of both organisational and clinical failure. We need to examine whether the way primary care is currently organised meets adequately the needs of multicultural communities, especially living in inner-city areas. There is very little understanding at present about the way minority ethnic groups in general and South Asian communities and other linguistic minorities interact with and access healthcare agencies at this level. South Asian communities also appear to be disadvantaged by the absence of strategic plans to improve community capacity in dealing with health matters as well as in the area of prevention or education. Once again, such failures only tend to enhance the sense of disempowerment and rejection experienced by the community when dealing with mental health problems. At the clinical level there is ample evidence that ethnicity of the patient has a direct impact on the assessment of psychological problems by the GP, irrespective of the ethnic background of the GP.[28] Very few GPs, for example, have training in cultural awareness and related skills and competency. These clinician characteristics are important in the assessment of people from cultural and ethnic minorities and, more so, in relation to the appraisal of psychological distress.

There could be several reasons for patients not to disclose their psychological distress to their GPs. Cultural minorities in particular might have a more sceptical view of the relevance of medical interventions in dealing with emotional or psychological problems. Interventions which are often offered, such as referral to mental health services or a diagnosis of mental illness, are often perceived as stigmatising, not culturally sanctioned (unlike physical illness) and/or irrelevant. While physical illness is typically conceived of as a personal affliction by Indian and Pakistani patients, emotional problems are intimately bound up with social roles.[35] Individually focused models of distress and psychotherapy may therefore be inapplicable. In the absence of suitable psychosocial interventions, it is possible that these differences in cultural language contribute both to the greater likelihood of Indian and Pakistani patients presenting with somatic symptoms[28] and to the higher proportion seeing a doctor.[27] It has been argued that pharmacological therapies are simply easier to deliver.[36] Certainly, the fact that only around one-third of Indian and Pakistani patients in our survey gave English as their preferred language demands that psychotherapists are recruited and trained who are able to converse with patients in the language with which they feel most comfortable. However, more fundamentally, we need to reflect on the appropriateness and acceptability of the services on offer.[37]

The preponderance of South Asian people with severe mental illness living in the family home suggests that there is a significant burden of care that is borne by the family. Often there is little acknowledgement of this within the formal system of mental healthcare and family-based interventions and support for carers are particularly lacking in relation to South Asian people with long-term mental health problems. Assumptions that the 'supposedly extended Asian family' is able to cope should be challenged[36] and non-institutionally based interventions promoted if Indian and Pakistani patients and their carers are to receive an equitable service. Nevertheless, caution is required before, for example, widely implementing family intervention programmes which are traditionally used in the management of schizophrenia. There is evidence that some of the models currently available for family interventions may not be as effective in Asian patients as for white patients, possibly because of the cultural specificity of concepts such as 'expressed emotion' which are used in such work.[38]

The rates of compulsory admission and satisfaction with inpatient services are not dissimilar across ethnic groups for first-episode schizophrenia. There is also evidence that the number of previous admissions is a significant predictor of dissatisfaction among younger black patients.[30] Service dissatisfaction and discordance, as well as disengagement from services, appear to emerge in the context of aversive and antagonistic experiences of psychiatric services. Early intervention programmes for people with psychotic disorders could therefore play a critical role in nurturing and sustaining more positive initial therapeutic relationships. Once a sequence of non-compliance–coercion–hostility becomes established, home treatment services, which may be more acceptable to minority ethnic groups,[39] similarly could offer a way to address the entrenched patterns of aversive hospital-based care encountered by South Asian populations. Primary care and community agencies as well as individual GPs have a major responsibility in ensuring that local mental health services are not only community based but are culturally appropriate to the needs of a diverse community.

Clearly, there is a pressing need to reappraise the way the NHS is responding to the mental healthcare needs of all minority ethnic groups. The experience of South Asian people at all levels in the care system, as well as in the general population, gives significant clues as to how we can improve the organisation and delivery of mental healthcare so that they suit the needs of this population. A national policy on ethnicity and mental health is long overdue and, four years after the publication of the Macpherson Report[6] and the imposition of statutory requirements to achieve race equality within the NHS, there are still significant delays and resistance to bringing about organisational reform and eradicating racism within the health service. However, reforms in these areas will not be sufficient by themselves to alter the mental health experience of people from South Asian communities and, indeed, that of other black and minority ethnic groups. Changes in professional practice, an understanding of the broader disadvantage affecting minority ethnic populations, an emphasis on cultural capability of clinicians and services, and a reappraisal of the theories and assumptions which underpin current psychiatric practice are all necessary before the current ethnic inequalities in service experience and outcome can be addressed adequately.

References

1   Bhopal R (1997) Is research into ethnicity and health racist, unsound, or important science? *BMJ*. **314**: 1751.

2   Ahmad WIU (1993) *'Race' and Health in Contemporary Britain.* Open University Press, Buckingham.

3   National Schizophrenia Fellowship (2000) *No Change: a report by the National Schizophrenia Fellowship comparing the experience of people from different ethnic groups who use mental health services.* NSF, London.

4   Sainsbury Centre For Mental Health (2002) *Breaking the Circles of Fear: a review of the relationship between mental health services and the African and Caribbean communities.* SCMH, London.

5   National Institute Of Mental Health In England (2003) *Inside Outside: improving mental health services for black and minority ethnic groups in England.* (www.nimhe.org.uk)

6   Macpherson W (1999) *The Stephen Lawrence Inquiry: report of an Inquiry by Sir William Macpherson of Cluny advised by Tim Cook, The Right Reverend Dr John Sentamu, Dr Richard Stone.* The Stationery Office, London.

7   Commission For Racial Equality (2002) *Code of Practice on the Duty to Promote Racial Equality.* CRE, London.

8   Erens B, Primatesta P and Prior G (2001) *Health Survey for England: the health of minority ethnic groups.* The Stationery Office, London.

9   Weich S and Lewis G (1998) Poverty, unemployment and common mental disorders: population-based cohort study. *BMJ.* **317**: 115–19.

10 Nazroo JY (1998) Genetic, cultural or socio-economic vulnerability? Explaining ethnic inequalities in health. *Sociology of Health and Illness.* **20**: 710–30.

11 Commander MJ, Sashidharan SP, Odell S *et al.* (1997) Access to mental health care in an inner-city health district. 1. Pathways into and within specialist psychiatric services. *British Journal of Psychiatry.* **170**: 312–16.

12 Weich S and Mcmanus S (2002) Common mental disorders. In: Sproston K and Nazroo J (eds) *Ethnic Minority Psychiatric Illness Rates in the Community (EMPIRIC).* National Centre for Social Research, London.

13 Stansfeld S and Sproston K (2002) Social support and networks. In: Sproston K and Nazroo J (eds) *Ethnic Minority Psychiatric Illness Rates in the Community (EMPIRIC).* National Centre for Social Research, London.

14 Nazroo J, Fenton S, Karlsen S *et al.* (2002) Context, cause and meaning: qualitative insights. In: Sproston K and Nazroo J (eds) *Ethnic Minority Psychiatric Illness Rates in the Community (EMPIRIC).* National Centre for Social Research, London.

15 Gee GC (2002) A multilevel analysis of the relationship between institutional and individual racial discrimination and health status. *American Journal of Public Health.* **92**: 615–23.

16 McKenzie K (2003) Racism and health. *BMJ.* **326**: 65–6.

17 Modood T, Berhoud R, Lakey J *et al.* (1997) *Ethnic Minorities in Britain: diversity and disadvantage. The Fourth National Survey of Ethnic Minorities.* Policy Studies Institute, London.

18 Clancy A, Hough M, Aust R *et al.* (2001) *Crime, Policing and Justice: the experience of ethnic minorities: Findings from the 2000 British Crime Survey.* Home Office, London.

19 Goldberg D and Huxley P (1992) *Common Mental Disorders.* Routledge, London.

20 Goldberg D and Williams P (1988) *A User's Guide to the General Health Questionnaire.* NFER-Nelson, Windsor.

21 Bhui K, Stansfeld S, Hull S *et al.* (2003) Ethnic variations in pathways to, and use of, specialist mental health services in the UK. Systematic review. *British Journal of Psychiatry.* **182**: 105–16.

22 Commander MJ, Sashidharan SP, Odell S *et al.* (1997) Access to mental health care in an inner-city health district. 2. Association with demographic factors. *British Journal of Psychiatry.* **170**: 317–20.

23 Spitzer RL, Williams JBW, Gibbon M *et al.* (1992) The structured clinical interview for DSM IIIR (SCID). 1. History, rationale and description. *Archives of General Psychiatry.* **49**: 624–9.

24 Husain N, Creed F and Tomenson B (1997) Adverse social circumstances and depression in people of Pakistani origin in the UK. *British Journal of Psychiatry.* **17**: 434–8.

25 Jacob KS, Bhugra D, Lloyd KR *et al.* (1998) Common mental disorders, explanatory models and consultation behaviour among Indian women living in the UK. *Journal of the Royal Society of Medicine.* **91**: 66–71.

26 Angermeyer MC, Matschinger R and Riedel-Heller SG (1999) Whom to ask for help in case of a mental disorder? Preferences of the lay public. *Social Psychiatry and Psychiatric Epidemiology.* **34**: 202–10.

27 Bhui K (1999) Common mental disorders among people with origins in, or immigrant from, India and Pakistan. *International Review of Psychiatry.* **4** (11): 136–44.

28 Odell S, Surtees PG, Wainwright NWJ *et al.* (1997) Determinants of general practitioner recognition of psychological problems in a multi-ethnic, inner-city health district. *British Journal of Psychiatry.* **171**: 537–41.

29 Commander MJ, Sashidharan SP, Odell S *et al.* (In press.) Characteristics of patients and patterns of psychiatric service use in ethnic minorities. *International Journal of Social Psychiatry.*

30 Commander MJ, Cochrane R, Sashidharan SP *et al.* (1999) Mental health care for Asian, black and white patients with non-affective psychoses: pathways to psychiatric hospital, in-patient and after care. *Social Psychiatry and Psychiatric Epidemiology.* **34** (9): 484–91.

31 Patel MG, Wright DJ, Jerwood D *et al.* (2002) Prescribing of lipid-lowering drugs to South Asian patients: ecological study. *BMJ.* **325**: 25–6.

32 Stewart A, Rao J, Osho-Williams G *et al.* (2002) Audit of primary care management of angina in Sandwell. *Journal of the Royal Society for the Promotion of Health.* **122**: 112–17.

33 Feder G, Cook AM, Magee P *et al.* (2002) Ethnic differences in invasive management of coronary disease: prospective study of patients undergoing angiography. *BMJ.* **324**: 511–16.

34 Mclean C, Campbell C and Cornish F (2003) African-Caribbean interactions with mental health services in the UK: experience and expectations of exclusion as (re)productive of health inequalities. *Social Science and Medicine.* **56**: 657–69.

35 Beliappa J (1991) *Illness or Distress? Alternative models of mental health.* Confederation of Indian Organisations, London.

36 Mercer K (1984) Black communities' experience of psychiatric services. *International Journal of Social Psychiatry.* **30**: 22–7.

37 Bhugra D (1997) Setting up psychiatric services: cross-cultural issues in planning and delivery. *International Journal of Social Psychiatry.* **41**: 242–56.

38 Hashemi AH and Cochrane R (1999) Expressed emotion and schizophrenia: a review of studies across cultures. *International Review of Psychiatry.* **11**: 219–24.

39 Sashidharan SP (1999) Alternatives to institutional psychiatry. In: Bhugra D and Bhal V (eds) *Ethnicity: an agenda for mental health.* Gaskell, London.

CHAPTER 9

Diabetes: a challenge for health professionals and policy makers

Dinesh Nagi

This chapter, by discussing diabetes, examines the implications for primary care of another specific condition. It specifically considers the challenges facing practitioners and policy makers arising from the high and rising prevalence of diabetes in South Asian people compared to the 'white' population. Although diabetes may present in different ways and includes type 1 and type 2 diabetes, discussion in this chapter will be limited to type 2 diabetes, which comprises more than 85 per cent of all people with diabetes. The chapter is in four sections. The first considers the 'burden' of diabetes and explores possible explanations for the high prevalence of diabetes among South Asian populations. The second section considers diabetes in the clinical context and discusses associated complications of diabetes as well as possible risk factors. The third part focuses on the question of whether we can improve clinical care for diabetes in South Asian people, and considers the arguments for improving access, understanding cultural perceptions, raising awareness and education. The potential impact of the new primary care trusts and National Service Framework for Diabetes is also explored. The final section discusses strategies for preventing diabetes and improving diabetes care in South Asian people.

This chapter has particular relevance to those working in primary care because, with a primary care-led NHS, much of diabetes care will be provided in the primary care environment, with more specialist intervention being provided by secondary care. Recent changes in the NHS, initiated by *The NHS Plan* (2000),[1] the recent establishment of PCTs and the publication of the diabetes NSF, means that the management of diabetes will become more community based with specialist general practitioners running community-based clinics supported by dieticians, podiatrists and diabetes specialist nurses. Several cities, for example, are developing such community-based clinics.

The prevalence of diabetes

Diabetes is a common disorder, and it is likely more than two million people in the UK have the condition. There are also considerable numbers who remain undiagnosed. Worldwide the prevalence of diabetes is expected to rise dramatically over the next 25 years. The biggest rise will be seen in countries such as India,

China and the USA and in populations with high prevalence of diabetes, such as migrant South Asians. Epidemiological studies of the prevalence of diabetes across various populations worldwide have provided interesting insights into the causes of diabetes and an analytical framework for examining the interaction between genetic and environmental influences.[2] In addition, studies of diabetes prevalence in South Asian populations have helped an understanding of the implications of both internal (within the same country) and external (into a different country) migration on diabetes.

In recent years evidence has accumulated which suggests that effective management of diabetes can reduce morbidity and mortality as well as reduce the chronic complications of the disease. In addition, it has become clear that effective management of diabetes requires active participation of patients, so that they feel empowered to develop skills to take control of their own lives. To develop and foster this self-care, development of the skills of the patient is essential and education remains a fundamental requirement to achieve this. Since diabetes is common among South Asian people living in the UK, it is appropriate to examine how this condition can be managed and outcomes improved, so that the heavy disease burden associated with the condition can be reduced.

Diabetes and South Asian people living in the UK

The first reports of high prevalence of diabetes in migrant South Asian populations came from Singapore and from the island of Fiji.[3] These studies suggested that diabetes in these migrant South Asian populations was three to four times more common than in the native populations. The first report focusing on diabetes among South Asian populations living in the UK came from the Southall Survey, which showed that diabetes in Southall was more prevalent in South Asian people when compared to European populations.[4] In 1985, a house-to-house survey of patients with known diabetes was carried out among 34 000 Asian and 27 000 European people. A total of 1143 subjects with diabetes were identified, of whom 761 were South Asians and 324 Europeans. The age-adjusted prevalence of diabetes in South Asian populations was 3.8 times higher compared with the European groups. Further, diabetes was five times more common in South Asian people between the ages of 40 and 64 years. The prevalence of diabetes increased with age: among those aged 50–59 prevalence was 8 per cent and for those aged 60–69 it was 12 per cent. Most South Asians in this study were Punjabi Sikhs from North India. The most interesting observation was that high prevalence of diabetes in South Asians was seen between the ages of 35 and 60 years and this was similar to that seen in Europeans, at both extremes of age. This would suggest that the major burden of diabetes in this community was among people of working age. This survey was designed to determine the number of people with a known diagnosis of diabetes, and was open to many difficulties and biases. Knowing, however, the lower access and utilisation of healthcare by South Asian communities, this study may have underestimated the true differences between South Asian and European populations, as diabetes may have remained undiagnosed in a higher proportion of South Asian people.

In another survey in the Foleshill area of Coventry, 4395 South Asian and 5508 European people were screened initially with measurement of random blood glucose as part of an initial screen for diagnosing diabetes.[5] Those who were found to have high blood glucose and a further random 10 per cent of subjects were assigned to have an oral glucose tolerance test (OGTT). Those with known diabetes (104 Europeans and 223 South Asians) were re-interviewed in more detail. The crude prevalence of diabetes was 3.2 per cent in European men compared to 12.4 per cent in South Asian men, and 4.7 per cent and 11.2 per cent for European and South Asian women respectively. This study also showed that the prevalence of impaired glucose tolerance (IGT), a category intermediate between normal glucose tolerance and diabetes, was also significantly higher in both South Asian men and women. South Asian populations, therefore, had high prevalence of diabetes. The results of these studies, on a background of a higher mortality from coronary heart disease in South Asians (see Chapter 7), highlighted a serious health issue among South Asian people. Some suggested that a considerable portion of the high mortality due to coronary heart disease in South Asian people could be explained by the higher prevalence of diabetes alone.[6]

Interestingly, subsequent studies from India also showed that diabetes was very common in native Indians living in India. Population surveys in South India as well as in Delhi have shown a prevalence of known diabetes that is comparable to that seen in South Asian people in the UK.[7] In the Delhi survey, the overall prevalence was 3.2 per cent and peaked at 16.9 per cent in the 60–64 age group. Diabetes was twice as common in men as in women. Further, 85 per cent of people with diabetes in this survey were businessmen and graduates with good socio-economic backgrounds, suggesting the influence of affluence on diabetes in India. In the survey from South India where an OGTT was performed to diagnose diabetes, the overall prevalence in this study, when adjusted for the age distribution of Indians living in London and Fiji, was 10 per cent and 9 per cent respectively.[8] Both these studies concluded that the prevalence of diabetes in different urban areas in India was comparable to the higher prevalence seen in South Asian people in the UK.

Why is diabetes more common in South Asian populations?

Initially it was thought that high rates of diabetes seen among South Asians in the UK might simply be due to the impact of migration to another country and as a consequence of the associated environmental factors or other as yet unidentified influences. Subsequent studies examined this hypothesis in more detail and reported that migration from a rural area to a nearby urban area within the same country produced a similar impact.[9] These observations would suggest that South Asian people are more susceptible to diabetes and that environmental factors associated with migration, be it an internal or external migration, are associated with high rates of diabetes.

It is now accepted that South Asians show insulin resistance (a reduced effectiveness of insulin in the body) syndrome and hyperinsulinaemia (high levels of insulin in the bloodstream) and that these play a crucial role in the development of diabetes. Insulin resistance appears to be a major contributing factor in the development of diabetes in this population. It is now clear that diabetes will only develop when beta cells can no longer compensate by producing enough insulin and a state of glucose intolerance develops, leading eventually to manifest diabetes (*see* Figure 9.1). Both insulin resistance and hyperinsulinaemia are believed to be the underlying cause of the metabolic syndrome in many populations world-wide as well as in South Asians.[10–13] This syndrome is characterised by several features, including obesity, physical inactivity, glucose intolerance, high blood pressure, abnormal lipids and coronary heart disease, in the same individuals (*see* Figure 9.2). There are no true population-based studies to determine the exact prevalence or incidence of type 2 diabetes in this population. It is accepted that the prevalence of diabetes in South Asian populations living in the UK, which include people of Indian, Pakistani and Bangladeshi origin, has been shown to be approximately three to six times more than that of European subjects.

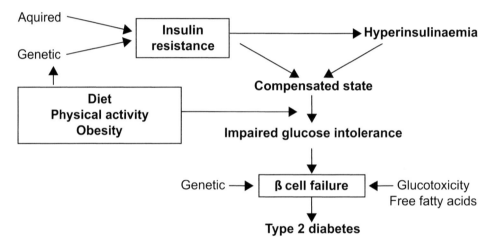

Figure 9.1   Pathogenesis of type 2 diabetes. It is believed that obesity, physical activity and genetic predisposition are causative factors and therefore contribute to the development of insulin resistance and hyperinsulinaemia. (PAI-1 = plasminogen activator inhibitor-1).

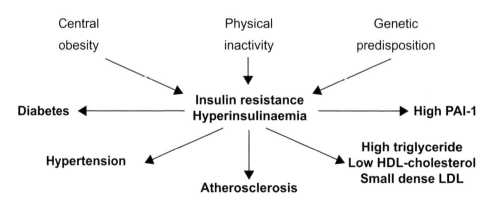

Figure 9.2   Characteristics of the metabolic syndrome (insulin resistance syndrome). Contribution of insulin resistance and beta cell dysfunction in type 2 diabetes. It shows that both insulin resistance and beta cell dysfunction are needed for the development of type 2 diabetes.

Studies in the mid-1980s showed that South Asian people had a greater level of insulin resistance than that seen in the white population. Several reports also confirmed high fasting insulin levels (a surrogate marker for insulin resistance), including our own studies, which used very highly specific assays for insulin, which only measure true insulin levels.[13,14] In addition it was also apparent that South Asian populations showed other important features of the metabolic syndrome, including central obesity and physical inactivity.[15,16] Studies confirmed that South Asian people show evidence of insulin resistance, hyperinsulinaemia and other features of the metabolic syndrome such as central obesity and physical inactivity more commonly than their European counterparts. It is also suggested that this ethnic group is more genetically susceptible to diabetes. However, more recently, an alternative hypothesis that low birth weight due to poor intrauterine nutrition may contribute to higher rates of diabetes has been advanced.[16]

Diabetes in the clinical context

Although the underlying nature of the disease in South Asian people is similar to that seen in the white population, there appear to be certain differences, which have been reported from various centres within the UK.[17,18] In the UK Prospective Diabetes Study (UKPDS), which recruited newly diagnosed patients with diabetes, there were 554 South Asian people included (372 males and 172 females). First, the onset of diabetes in this population occurs at a younger age: the mean age at diagnosis was 46.8 years in South Asian men and 47.6 years in South Asian women, while it was 51.8 years and 52.9 years in white men and women respectively.[19] This study also showed that in comparison with their white counterparts, South Asian people were significantly shorter and had lower body mass index (BMI). Despite this they had higher waist-to-hip circumference ratio, suggesting an element of central obesity.

This study also confirmed that the prevalence of peripheral vascular disease (shown by absent foot pulses) was significantly lower in South Asian people and this agreed with previously published data. The prevalence of high blood pressure was also lower in South Asian people. Similarly, the proportion of South Asian people taking blood pressure-lowering medication was lower. Moreover, South Asian people had significantly lower systolic and diastolic blood pressure in both sexes. South Asian men and women had significantly lower BMI yet higher waist-to-hip ratio, suggesting a more central distribution of fat. A significantly higher proportion of South Asian men and women led a sedentary life.

In addition, a positive family history is seen more often, suggesting a familial basis of diabetes. South Asian people also require insulin treatment at a much younger age. The UKPDS study showed that in relation to their disease management they would appear to respond similarly to lifestyle interventions, oral drug treatment and insulin treatment compared to their white counterparts. Our own studies have shown that South Asian people responded to metformin treatment in a similar fashion to white people.[20]

Complications of diabetes

South Asian people with or without diabetes are more likely than their white counterparts to develop premature coronary heart disease and their mortality rates have been shown to be higher, although recently published data from the UKPDS contradict these findings.[21] The risks of peripheral vascular disease and leg amputation seem to be comparatively much lower.[22] A study which included a large number of subjects, published recently, has reconfirmed this notion, showing that South Asian people have a quarter of the risk of white people.[23] These low rates were largely explained by low rates of peripheral vascular disease and neuropathy and in part by low rates of smoking. The reasons behind protection from peripheral vascular disease and neuropathy remain unknown.

Secondly, microalbuminuria and end-stage renal failure have been reported to be more pronounced in this population but interestingly they seem to have less retinopathy, another classic microvascular complication of diabetes, frequently associated with nephropathy. The rates of smoking in South Asians from India have been reported to be low except in people from Bangladesh, and this population appears to be less physically active compared to the white population. Studies examining the risk factors for diabetes in this population are few, but age, obesity, physical inactivity, a positive family history of diabetes and a previous history of gestational diabetes are all important.

Improving clinical care for South Asian populations

To have a real chance of improving the health of South Asians in relation to diabetes, we need to examine and understand the possible factors that may be associated with, or contribute to, some of the poor outcomes.

Diabetes remaining underdiagnosed

Although there is no systematic data suggesting that diabetes in this population is underdiagnosed, it would appear to be diagnosed at a later stage in South Asians compared to the white population. In the Coventry survey, the proportion of people who had undiagnosed diabetes was similar among South Asian and white people, but South Asian people with new diabetes were more symptomatic at the time of diagnosis of their diabetes.[24] This suggests that these subjects may have had diabetes which remained undiagnosed for a longer period of time than white people. If this were to be the case, one would have expected to find higher prevalence of diabetes complications at the time of diagnosis, but this appears not to be the case, as observed in the UKPDS.[25]

Access to healthcare

Studies have suggested that poor outcome related to diabetes may be due to poor access to healthcare.[26] There are no good qualitative health studies exploring the underlying reasons for this. Unless this kind of information is available, it will prove extremely difficult to put systems in place to improve access to healthcare for these individuals. Suggestions have been made that poor access may be related to ignorance about the disease and its outcomes or other socio-economic reasons, which should be open to intervention and manipulation by better access to information and education.

Cultural differences in the perception of chronic diseases

Many health professionals believe that South Asian people have a different understanding of the concept of chronic diseases, which are lifelong and require continual medical supervision and therapy. Applying this thinking to diabetes is inappropriate and at times can lead to some serious consequences. Some patients (despite being given adequate explanations) may seek alternative medical help, with the misguided notion or belief that there will be some 'magic' cure available which is beyond the grasp of modern science. The general population seems to hold similar perceptions. Nonetheless, this often means they discontinue ongoing medical treatments, with consequent poor control of diabetes and related problems, in the belief that their diabetes will improve with other alternative treatments.

Lack of tested educational models

To date, little if any efforts have been made to understand and develop educational interventions that are culture-specific to South Asian people. To assume that producing patient information leaflets in different South Asian languages can be equated to a culturally bound intervention is not only naïve but foolish (see also Chapter 2). This kind of approach is highly unlikely to empower South Asian communities and individuals. To think that interventions which may be effective for European patients with diabetes will work equally well or even work at all for South Asians is untested and, therefore, undesirable. There is little or no information on the barriers to care in these populations. The issue as to how social or family support, or the lack of it, will impact on the diabetes care in these populations remains largely unknown.

Potential impact of primary care organisations and the National Service Framework for Diabetes

The NHS is going through a major modernisation process, which includes recognition that primary care has a leading role to play in the delivery of high-quality healthcare. As we have seen, this has meant reorganisation within primary care and the formation of PCTs. In addition, the government has launched its agenda of NSFs for common diseases, which includes diabetes. How this will impact on healthcare for ethnic groups such as South Asians remains to be seen. One of the main aims of the NSF is to address and remove the inequalities in relation to diabetes care and also improve overall quality. Therefore, one is hopeful that the opportunity provided by the diabetes NSF will be grasped by those close to delivering healthcare to these populations, and care pathways will be established for provision of better diabetes care. We have already seen, for example, how successful services for those with heart disease have been developed by PCTs in response to the NSF for Coronary Heart Disease.

Do we know how to manage diabetes in South Asians?

As far as the management of diabetes in South Asian populations is concerned, there are very few studies that examine this issue in detail. It is now agreed that the outcomes in relation to certain disease-specific and patient-specific indicators would appear to be much less satisfactory in South Asian populations. Whether these differences in health outcomes are due to poor rates of uptake of healthcare or due to cultural and sociological differences remains speculative. South Asian people in the UK have been treated for their diabetes using the same model of care designed for the indigenous white populations. Chapter 2 outlined the problems inherent in such an approach. No specific efforts have been made to understand the real fundamental barriers to the provision of diabetes care to South Asian people. These barriers could be of a personal nature, including health beliefs, cultural and language barriers, community barriers, issues of trust and understanding between this population and the healthcare providers, and psychosocial barriers.[27]

How we make progress and move forward to improve diabetes care in this population remains a topic of debate among health policy makers and health professionals who are involved in providing care for these ethnic groups. Clear strategies need to be developed for provision of care for people with diabetes in this population and these should include:

- South Asian people need to be involved in the development of the local diabetes service
- a strategy for improving care in these ethnic groups requires the development and delivery of an innovative, culturally sensitive, educational programme to raise the awareness of the implications of having diabetes
- such strategies may need to include training more ethnic minority physicians and educators who are more likely to engender a feeling of trust and cultural understanding between patients and the healthcare professionals
- these strategies should also include efforts not only at secondary prevention of diabetic complications, but also to look at the population as a whole to improve their health in general
- understanding that poor health outcomes are related to poor socio-economic status and including in any strategy specific efforts to prevent the disease. An example of this could be publicity campaigns delivered in the relevant languages using appropriate media (South Asian television channels, radio, newspapers and books)
- developing easy screening methods for early detection of diabetes to minimise risk of complications and subsequent morbidity
- developing structured and co-ordinated diabetes care which incorporates cultural sensitivity for this population.

Prevention of diabetes in South Asians

Diabetes is a preventable disease and the risk can be reduced by lifestyle interventions and drug treatment.[27] Interventions aimed at people who are at high risk of diabetes are being successfully tested for effective methods of prevention. It is easy to screen and find those at risk of diabetes by simple and reliable tests.[28] Of the published literature on prevention of diabetes, three randomised studies are worth considering here. In a Chinese study, the first properly conducted randomised study to be performed, the risk of diabetes was reduced by diet, diet and exercise and exercise alone.[29] The Da-Qing study from China was a population-based randomised study. A total of 576 subjects with IGT were randomised to four groups (control, diet alone, exercise alone or both) and were followed for an average period of 5.6 years. The incidence of diabetes was reduced equally, by 50 per cent, in all three intervention groups. Some general points of interest emerged from this first properly randomised and controlled intervention study.

- Lifestyle interventions in the form of diet and physical activity for up to six years significantly reduced the development of diabetes.
- The effects of diet or exercise were similar: both reduced the risk of diabetes.
- The risk of diabetes was reduced despite fairly modest reduction in body weight (approximately 2 kg).
- The increase in physical activity was modest but sustained over the lifetime of the study.
- The effects were similar in obese and non-obese subjects.

The results of this intervention trial cannot be generalised to other ethnic groups and need to be replicated in other ethnic groups with a high risk of developing diabetes.

The results of a recently published study from Finland have been extremely encouraging.[30] In this study, 522 middle-aged subjects (172 men, 350 women) with a mean age of 55 and with a mean BMI of 31 received an intervention consisting of individual counselling to reduce weight, decrease saturated fat intake, increase fibre intake and increase physical activity. After an average follow-up of 3.2 years, subjects in the intervention group lost 4.2 kg of weight compared to 0.8 kg in the control group at year 1 and 3.5 kg and 0.8 kg respectively at year 2. The cumulative incidence of diabetes in the intervention group was 11 per cent (95 per cent confidence interval (CI) 6–15) compared to 23 per cent (95 per cent CI 17–29) in the control group. Lifestyle interventions, therefore, resulted in a total risk reduction of 58 per cent; results which were highly significant. Further, the reduced incidence of diabetes was related to changes in lifestyle. To interpret data in another way, 22 subjects with IGT (i.e. at high risk of future diabetes) will need to be treated for one year (or five subjects for five years) in this way to prevent one case of diabetes.

A large multicentre study, the Diabetes Prevention Project (DPP), has recently reported its findings. The DPP set out to recruit 4000 subjects at high risk of type 2 diabetes.[31] In this study, eligibility criteria included: age > 25 years, minimal overweight and IGT as defined by World Health Organization (WHO) criteria. This study included 50 per cent women and up to 50 per cent of subjects who were non-white. Twenty-five per cent of subjects were also over 65 years. Intensive lifestyle interventions were tested along with drug interventions to modify insulin resistance. Subjects were randomised according to diet and exercise or use of the drug metformin. The results of this study confirmed that diabetes could be prevented by lifestyle modifications and by drug interventions. The risk of diabetes was reduced by both lifestyle changes in the form of diet and exercise and also by metformin treatment.[32] After an average follow-up of 2.8 years, the incidence of diabetes was 11.0, 7.8 and 4.8 cases per 100 person-years of follow-up in placebo, metformin and lifestyle interventions respectively. The lifestyle intervention reduced diabetes incidence by 58 per cent and metformin by 38 per cent, compared to placebo treatment. The results of this trial were similar in men, women and in all ethnic groups studied. Moreover, lifestyle interventions were equally effective in younger and older individuals.

At present there are no published studies from Indian, Pakistani or Bangladeshi populations of intervention to prevent diabetes in their respective countries. It would appear to be an attractive option in a population with high prevalence of diabetes, such as South Asian Indians, as the rates of diabetes are projected to double over the next 20 years.[33] It remains for policy makers to make this a public health issue and urgent intervention trials are needed in these populations. It needs to be remembered, however, that lifestyle interventions in different ethnic groups may be particularly challenging,[34] suggesting that when intervening with lifestyle measures, different strategies may need to be adopted for different ethnic groups. In a study reported from Tanzania in people of Hindu religion, simple dietary advice to eat less and exercise more by walking for 30 minutes per day resulted in protection from progression to diabetes.[35] In most studies of lifestyle interventions, there was a tendency towards a reduction in risk factors for cardiovascular disease such as total and low density lipoprotein (LDL)-cholesterol, triglyceride and a decrease in systolic and diastolic blood pressure.

Conclusion

In summary, diabetes in South Asian people is an important health issue which needs urgent attention. We should strive to gather evidence about strategies that work in reducing the disease burden on this population. Both primary and secondary prevention of diabetes are of crucial importance in this population at very high risk of diabetes and coronary heart disease. In the new primary care-led NHS, PCTs, by forming local partnerships, can offer opportunities to develop strategies, guided by the diabetes NSF, to improve care for their local communities.

References

1   Department of Health (2002) *The NHS Plan*. HMSO, London.
2   Knowler WC, McCance DR, Nagi DK *et al.* (1993) Epidemiological studies of the causes of diabetes mellitus. In: Leslie RDG (ed) *Causes of Diabetes*, pp. 187–218. John Wiley & Sons, Chichester.
3   Cassidy JT (1967) Diabetes in Fiji. *New Zealand Medical Journal.* **66**: 167–72.
4   Mather HM and Keen H (1985) The Southall Diabetic Survey: prevalence of known diabetes in Asians and Europeans. *BMJ.* **291**: 1081–4.
5   Simmons D, Williams DRR and Powell MJ (1989) Prevalence of diabetes in a predominantly Asian community: preliminary findings of the Coventry Diabetes Study. *BMJ.* **298**: 18–21.
6   Woods KL, Samanta A and Burden AC (1989) Diabetes mellitus as a risk factor for myocardial infarction in Asians and Europeans. *British Heart Journal.* **62**: 118–22.

7   Verma NPS, Mehta SP, Madhu S *et al.* (1986) Prevalence of known diabetes in an urban Indian environment: the Darya Ganj Diabetes Survey. *BMJ.* **293**: 423–4.

8   Ramachandran A, Jali MV, Mohan V *et al.* (1988) High prevalence of diabetes in an urban population in South India. *BMJ.* **297**: 587–90.

9   Ramachandran A, Snehalatha C, Dharamraj D *et al.* (1992) Prevalence of glucose intolerance in Asian Indians. Urban–rural differences and significance of upper body adiposity. *Diabetes Care.* **15**: 1348–55.

10   Greenhalgh PM (1997) Diabetes in British South Asians: nature, nurture, and culture. *Diabetic Medicine.* **14**: 10–18.

11   Knowler WC, Pettitt DJ, Saad MF *et al.* (1990) Diabetes mellitus in the Pima Indians: incidence, risk factors and pathogenesis. *Diabetes/Metabolism Review.* **6**: 1–27.

12   Ramachandran A, Snehalatha C, Visvanathan V *et al.* (1997) Risk of NIDDM conferred by obesity and central adiposity in different ethnic groups: a comparative analysis between Asian Indians, Mexican Americans and Whites. *Diabetes Research and Clinical Practice.* **36**: 121–5.

13   Nagi DK, Mohamed-Ali V, Walji S *et al.* (1996) Hyperinsulinaemia and insulin resistance syndrome – a comparison of Caucasian and Asian subjects using specific assays for insulin, intact proinsulin and des 31,32 proinsulin. *Diabetes Care.* **19**: 39–42.

14   Nagi DK, Knowler WC, Mohamed Ali V *et al.* (1998) Intact proinsulin, des 31,32 proinsulin and specific insulin concentrations among non-diabetic and diabetic subjects in populations at varying risk of type II diabetes. *Diabetes Care.* **21**: 127–33.

15   McKeigue PM, Shah B and Marmot MG (1991) Relation of central obesity and insulin resistance with high diabetes prevalence and cardiovascular risk in South Asians. *Lancet.* **337**: 382–6.

16   Knight TM, Smith Z, Whittles A *et al.* (1992) Insulin resistance, diabetes, and risk markers for ischaemic heart disease in Asian men and non-Asian men in Bradford. *British Heart Journal.* **67**: 343–50.

17   Hales CN and Barker DJP (1992) Type 2 (non-insulin dependent) diabetes mellitus: the thrifty phenotype hypothesis. *Diabetologia.* **35**: 595–601.

18   Feltbower RG, Bodansky HJ, McKinney PA *et al.* (2002) Trends in the incidence of childhood diabetes in South Asians and other children in Bradford, UK. *Diabetic Medicine.* **19**: 162–7.

19   UK Prospective Diabetes Study XII (1994) Differences between Asian, Afro-Caribbean and white Caucasian type 2 diabetic patients at diagnosis of diabetes. *Diabetic Medicine.* **11**: 670–8.

20   Nagi DK and Yudkin JS (1993) The effects of metformin on insulin resistance, risk factors for cardiovascular disease and plasminogen activator inhibitor (PAI-1) in non-insulin-dependent (NIDDM) subjects: a study of two ethnic groups. *Diabetes Care.* **16**: 621–9.

21   UKPDS 32 (1998) Ethnicity and cardiovascular disease: the incidence of myocardial infarction in white, South Asian and Afro-Caribbean patients with type 2 diabetes. *Diabetes Care.* **352**: 837–65.

22   Gujral JS, McNally PG, O'Malley BP *et al.* (1993) Ethnic differences in the incidence of lower extremity amputation secondary to diabetes mellitus. *Diabetic Medicine.* **10**: 271–4.

23   Chaturvedi N, Abbott CA, Whally A *et al.* (2002) Risk of diabetes-related amputations in South Asians vs. Europeans in the UK. *Diabetic Medicine.* **19**: 99–104.

24   Simmons D and Powell MJ (1993) Metabolic and clinical characteristics of South Asians and Europeans in Coventry. *Diabetic Medicine.* **10**: 751–8.

25   UKPDS (1997) Effect of age at diagnosis and tissue damage during the first six years of NIDDM. *Diabetes Care.* **20**: 1435–41.

26   Hawthorne K (1994) Accessibility and use of health care services in the British Asian community. *Family Practice.* **11**: 453–9.

27   Simmonds D, Weblemoe T, Voyle J *et al.* (1998) Personal barriers to diabetes care: lessons from a multi-ethnic community in New Zealand. *Diabetic Medicine.* **15**: 958–64.

28   Knowler WC, Narayan KMV, Hanson RL *et al.* (1995) Perspective in diabetes: preventing non-insulin-dependent diabetes. *Diabetes.* **44**: 483–8.

29   Pan X, Li G, Hu Y *et al.* (1997) Effects of diet and exercise in preventing NIDDM in people with impaired glucose tolerance. *Diabetes Care.* **20**: 537–44.

30   Tuomilehto J, Lindstrom J, Eriksson JG *et al.* (2001) Prevention of type 2 diabetes mellitus by changes in lifestyle among subjects with impaired glucose tolerance. *New England Journal of Medicine.* **344**: 1343–50.

31   The Diabetes Prevention Program Research Group (1999) The Diabetes Prevention Program: design and methods for a clinical trial in the prevention of type 2 diabetes. *Diabetes Care.* **22**: 623–34.

32   The Diabetes Prevention Program Research Group (2001) Reduction in the incidence of type 2 diabetes with lifestyle intervention or metformin. *New England Journal of Medicine.* **346**: 393–403.

33   Narayan KMV, Hoskin M, Kozak D *et al.* (1998) Randomised clinical trial of lifestyle interventions in Pima Indians – a pilot study. *Diabetic Medicine* **15**: 66–72.

34   Ramaya KL, Swai ABM, Alberti KGMM *et al.* (1992) Lifestyle changes decrease rates of glucose intolerance and cardiovascular (CVD) risk factors: a six-year intervention study in a high-risk Hindu Indian sub-community. *Diabetologia.* **35** (Suppl. 1): A60.

35   King H and Rewers M (1993) WHO Ad Hoc Reporting Group. Global estimates for the prevalence of diabetes mellitus and impaired glucose tolerance in adults. *Diabetes Care.* **16**: 157–77.

PART 4

Implications for policy and practice

Better knowledge, better care and better outcomes: implications for primary care policy and practice

Shahid Ali

The previous chapters, by presenting a mix of theoretical and empirical debates, provide an understanding of ethnicity and primary care. We began by arguing for the need for an initial framework that integrated mainstream debates about ethnicity and health with an exploration of the current organisational changes occurring in primary care. We then looked at specific policy examples, such as clinical governance, user involvement and partnership, to explore primary care's relationship to South Asian populations, before considering three 'disease-specific' case studies which reflect current NHS priorities. In doing so, we have outlined the disadvantage experienced by South Asian populations and the difficulties faced by primary care as it struggles to promote and provide more equitable and accessible care.

Understanding the process and outcome of disadvantage, as Chapter 2 demonstrated, is different from doing something about it. Focusing on the needs of South Asian populations is not the same as responding to those needs. Disadvantage and discrimination are not inevitable and we need to use our increasing knowledge base to transform service provision and provide better primary care for South Asian populations. To achieve change requires debates around ethnicity and primary care to be high on the ever-increasing agenda of primary care. Debates about ethnicity and primary care and the resultant clarity of information and purpose can enable primary care to address the current concerns of how and why the organisation and delivery of primary care have failed to understand and implement changes needed to improve care for South Asian populations. Such debates could be used to challenge, promote and support informed, achievable and 'real' changes at the 'front line'.

To do this, primary care needs to be more flexible and sensitive to the needs of South Asian populations. But before this, primary care has to learn how to engage with South Asian populations, to deal with issues such as poor communication, cultural difference and the attitudes of health professionals, which can often act against the involvement of South Asian users. Without a successful and concerted effort to involve South Asian users, primary care cannot begin to understand the needs of South Asian populations and make meaningful changes in the way services are provided. At the same time, we also need to understand how primary care is being reorganised (*see* Chapter 3). The recent radical changes in the NHS have placed primary care into a more central and leading role than ever before (see Department of Health, 2001 and 2002).[1,2] The resultant restructuring of the NHS, as we have seen, has created primary care trusts, which serve a smaller area and more defined communities of patients than the previous health authorities. This provides opportunities to allow the needs of the local communities to be determined, assessed and addressed in a clearer and more robust way than ever before.

A recent analysis of the impact of this radical change on organisational culture and decision making has identified significant areas in which improvements still need to be made.[3] These changes, however, do provide an impetus to address some of the inadequacies of the existing system, thereby creating the potential for radical opportunities.[4] A major initiative, the introduction of clinical governance, ensures that primary care responds to the quality agenda as robustly as possible (*see* Chapter 4). Further, National Service Frameworks by introducing clearly stated objectives – in specific clinical domains – support the impetus for change and can act as drivers for enhancing quality of care (see Chapters 7, 8 and 9).[5–7] Driving up the quality agenda by introducing more accountability, achievable targets, financial rewards and better working conditions should help to empower primary care in the longer term, although it may also feel overwhelmed by continual change and having to meet numerous national targets.

Primary care trusts are statutory bodies, which have to respond to national priorities and determine, assess and address local priorities. Any PCT serving a large South Asian population is likely to face a high risk of coronary heart disease and, therefore, must introduce measures to tackle this issue. PCTs are further expected to reach certain 'quality markers' as defined by the Department of Health, as well as being performance managed by strategic health authorities and assessed by the Commission for Health Improvement. Ethnicity must inform the basis of such performance management and assessments of PCTs' activities.

This reorganisation of primary care presents several opportunities for introducing ideas about equity and equality into the fabric of primary care organisations before organisational re-annealing occurs. PCTs, for example, now have financial resources which can be utilised to enable better communication by providing adequate language support in primary care. This, as Chapter 2 demonstrated, has been shown to empower the patient and prevent misunderstandings, myths and stereotypes. Better communication would also help primary care practitioners to understand the health needs, culture, lifestyles, social customs and religious practices of South Asian patients,[8] particularly since, as we have seen, practitioners often feel ill-equipped to deal with the demands of cultural and ethnic diversity, which further deprives South Asian people of their rights to services.

The challenge facing primary care

The challenges of delivering good quality care, overcoming communication difficulties and understanding cultural difference are not insurmountable. But how can primary care organisations make use of better knowledge to provide better care? In the first instance, PCTs need to engage with South Asian populations to ensure that their perspectives and needs adequately inform service delivery, rather than racist myths and stereotypes. Primary care also needs to better understand the emerging evidence base on inequalities and particularly the relationship between ethnicity and other forms of disadvantage. The treatment of South Asian populations as a homogenous group is not sustainable and any established policy and practice must be flexible in order to accommodate diversity and difference. Chapter 2, for example, argued against essentialised notions of ethnicity and suggested we needed to understand ethnic diversity within the broader context of socio-economic, gender, geographical and age difference, whereas Chapter 7 showed the complex relationship between ethnic origin and social class when making sense of rates of heart disease.

The comprehensive evidence base that already exists can be used to understand the difference in outcomes between the general and South Asian populations. Moreover, it can also be used to understand the barriers which need to be overcome to enhance the quality and care delivery to South Asian populations in primary care. In the quest for better knowledge there is a need for primary care to reconcile the theoretical debates on ethnicity and health and the emerging empirical evidence base, and ground the emerging insights in the 'reality' of primary care organisational development, policy and everyday practice. As practitioners, we regularly see research evidence, sometimes conflicting, from sources such as journals, books, the Web, guidelines and national and PCT directives. But how do we begin to make sense of all this evidence, let alone think through the specifics of the relationship of the evidence to South Asian populations? Chapter 3 touched on some of the dilemmas faced by primary care practitioners in their use of research evidence.

Evidence compiled by the Department of Health not only has to be implemented by the PCTs, but is also used to assess their performance. Given that PCTs have defined and manageable populations, this provides the necessary environment to determine the needs of the local population through user involvement, engaging with the local community as well as using audited information of quality and activity of care, provided at practice level. Such local intelligence and knowledge can be incorporated into policy in the Professional Executive Committee (PEC) and ratified by the PCT board. In this way the organisation can collect knowledge which reflects the needs of the immediate PCT population and takes responsibility at the highest level within the organisation, rather than relying on one appointed worker; a particular problem when dealing with ethnicity.[8] The policy once implemented can then be subject to, and driven by, clinical governance to ensure delivery and quality standards.

It is also imperative that PCTs responsible for providing and commissioning care for a majority South Asian population have a representative PEC and board, with adequate numbers of senior managers and professionals from the South Asian community, who can provide the local intelligence needed to ensure that better knowledge of and changes to services are not sidelined but that these changes are implemented robustly to bring about better care outcomes. Such individuals can ensure that more appropriate polices for South Asians are developed and that the needs of South Asian populations are not misrepresented by a failure to engage with cultural differences or by thinking that the problems are too difficult to solve, such as the need for language support.[3]

In achieving such an organisation shift, it is essential that issues such as diversity and equality should not be considered as 'soft' issues which can be left lower down or even off the agenda because managers are far too busy (see Atkin,

2003 for a broader discussion of the consequences of this view).[4] This can be prevented by raising awareness of different cultures, removing ignorance and reducing discriminatory practices. This would also make the PCT more attractive to potential employees from diverse backgrounds and should help to retain staff who are committed to and enthusiastic about making positive change. PCTs which recruit individuals from the local community in an open and fair way are in a better position to provide more accessible, culturally and religiously sensitive services valued by the users. Moreover, it should be remembered that by refusing to engage with this agenda, PCTs could incur significant human and legal costs for the organisation.[9] As we have seen, the Commission for Racial Equality is keen to ensure that the provisions outlined in the amendments to the 1976 Race Relations Act are reflected in the organisational practices of public organisations, and are prepared to take legal action against those organisations who ignore the Act (see Chapter 2).

Improving outcomes in heart disease: a case study

There are successful models found in the UK where the use of better knowledge has led to changes in policy and to greater understanding of culture and difference, thereby facilitating changes in service delivery and improving outcomes for South Asian populations. If we take coronary heart disease (CHD) as an example, we can see that the evidence base is considerable and complex. PCTs and primary care practitioners may hold the notion that all South Asian people exhibit the same risks for CHD, despite this being questioned by the rising body of evidence. In the chapter on CHD it has been shown that as well as migration histories of Indians, Pakistanis and Bangladeshis being different, the detail of their individual cultural identities is different too (*see* Chapter 7). The socio-economic positions of different subgroups within the South Asian population are quite distinct in terms of risk for heart disease, and socio-economic position is indeed an underlying risk factor which could explain much of the observed ethnic difference. We also know that rates of heart disease do rise and fall in different populations although why this happens is not, at present, clear. Considering some examples of how work in primary care has engaged South Asian people may help us to understand the process by which underlying causes of CHD, such as poor socio-economic position, experiences of racism, discrimination in the provision of services and poor access to care, result in heart disease. It is, therefore, important to consider multifactorial explanations for the higher rate of CHD in all communities, including South Asian populations. Explanations that emphasise only one risk factor may not identify the inter-relationships between different risk factors.

Consequently, a PCT strategy to reduce the risk of heart disease in South Asian populations needs to have elements of primary and secondary prevention as well as a social dimension. This would allow the inter-relationship between genetic, biological and environmental factors to be appropriately considered.

Prior to the radical change in the NHS, some argued that the high rates of heart disease amongst South Asian populations in Britain required a nationwide coronary health programme. This programme needed to be specifically tailored to the needs of South Asian populations and religious and community leaders had to help by raising the awareness of modifiable risk factors for CHD amongst the communities.[10] It has also been suggested that such a programme could be organised through places of worship, community centres, schools and by using the ethnic media. Further, such a policy argued that general practices serving large South Asian populations should provide separate clinics to modify risks for CHD in South Asian people. So far though, perhaps through ignorance or a deliberate failure to engage with the complex difference seen amongst South Asian populations, the same services appear to be provided according to 'white norms' which clearly cannot recognise difference and diversity and where assumptions have been made that services are equally appropriate for everyone (*see* Chapter 2). However, the new primary care-led NHS allows opportunities for closer working between communities and local primary healthcare teams. This would enable PCTs, with the support of local communities, to develop a joint strategy which can address issues of awareness, education, language and risk reduction in a more coherent and systematic way. Further, taking the current national NHS strategy to its conclusion should mean questioning the distinction between medical and social care, which would provide the impetus to reduce some of the socio-economic factors which contribute to ill health and inequality.

A successful example adopted by one Leicester PCT has combined primary care and community health promotion to reduce risk factors for CHD in South Asian populations.[11] The objective of this project was to improve primary and secondary prevention of heart disease in general practices that had high levels of South Asian patients. There were several strands to the project. These involved the development and subsequent implementation of a training and awareness programme for health professionals, a secondary prevention programme for general practice, a public awareness campaign and a peer education programme for the South Asian community. This project has been very successful in engaging and driving changes in primary care to help improve management of CHD. A community education programme was also developed. To ensure its success the local PCT adopted it, and this shows how PCTs working in a defined population base coupled with clear guidance provided in the NSF for Coronary Heart Disease can allow local solutions to be developed to prevent heart disease. Such projects also require 'local champions' who not only understand the problems and needs but also can position themselves to influence change that is evidence based and shows better outcomes.

Other PCTs have similarly developed local solutions for heart disease. Bradford South and West PCT has developed nurse-led primary care clinics in each of the practices to improve both primary and secondary prevention of heart disease. This strategy has allowed a more systematic approach to reducing heart disease by ensuring call and recall systems are established and closely monitoring risks for heart disease, including smoking, high blood pressure, diet, poor activity, cholesterol and adherence to medication to reduce risk and to prevent mortality. This PCT has also now started working with schools to raise awareness of primary prevention of heart disease at the earliest possible stage so that positive messages that encourage prevention can be delivered early.

Conclusion

There are several challenges facing primary care that need to be overcome before we can achieve better care outcomes for South Asian populations living in the UK.

Strategies need to be broad based and inclusive. This requires an approach that takes cultural and religious sensitivities into account, while at the same time remaining flexible to account for heterogeneity within South Asian populations. Methods of raising awareness need an effective communication and dissemination strategy using appropriate media to raise awareness and engage the user. Considering the communities at large, their perspectives and cultural wishes as well as religious and health beliefs, can help develop flexible primary care provision.

In order to address the underlying causes of ill health in South Asian populations, such as poor socio-economic position, experiences of racism, discrimination in the provision of services and poor access, PCTs need to be inclusive, tolerant and understanding and take up the challenge of understanding difference and diversity in South Asian populations. Active community participation can inform services and ensure adequate language support and sensitive and culturally aware staff (see Chapters 4, 5 and 6). PCTs must also adopt innovative ways to deliver education and information, using video and audio-tapes if needed, which will support flexible, customised mainstream services. More generally, examples of good practice do exist and we need to ensure these are known about and inform service development, particularly since there is a tendency to describe disadvantage and discrimination rather than do anything about it.

PCTs have been provided with financial resources and decision-making capabilities that can support such initiatives. To this end, PCTs should use their new-found power to establish a diverse management structure, produce coherent strategies based on better knowledge and provide high-quality services which result in better care and lead to better outcomes for South Asian populations. Disadvantage is not inevitable and we need to apply our growing evidence base, while taking advantage of the opportunities provided by organisation change, to secure accessible and appropriate primary care for South Asian people.

References

1   Department of Health (2001) *Shifting the Balance of Power within the NHS.* HMSO, London.
2   Department of Health (2002) *The NHS Plan.* HMSO, London.
3   Ali R (2003) *An Analysis of the Strategy for Radical Change in the NHS: the experience in Bradford, West Yorkshire.* (MBA dissertation.) Bradford University, Bradford.
4   Atkin K (2003) Health care in South Asian populations: making sense of policy and practice. In: Sayyid B, Ali N and Singh VK (eds) *Asian Nation: postcolonial settlers in Britain.* Hurst, London.
5   Department of Health (1999) *National Service Framework for Mental Health.* HMSO, London.
6   Department of Health (2000) *National Service Framework for Coronary Heart Disease.* HMSO, London.
7   Department of Health (2003) *National Service Framework for Diabetes.* HMSO, London.
8   Anionwu E and Atkin K (2001) *The Politics of Sickle Cell and Thalassaemia.* Open University Press, Buckingham.

9   Weston D and Welsh A (2003) Chapter and diverse. *Health Services Journal.*
    113(5853): 30.

10 Gupta S, de Belder A and O'Hughes L (1995) Avoiding premature coronary
    deaths in Asians in Britain: spend now on prevention or pay later for
    treatment. *BMJ.* **311**: 1035–6.

11 Stevenson K, Baker R, Farooqi A *et al.* (2001) Features of primary health care
    teams associated with success and quality improvement of diabetes care:
    a qualitative study. *Family Practice.* **18** (1): 21–6.

Index